Awakened Cuisine

Vibrant plant-based recipes
from our island café

Koh Phangan, Thailand

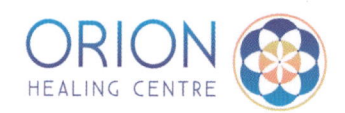

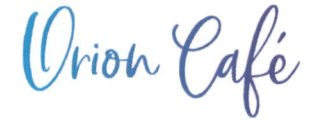

ORION HEALING CENTRE   Orion Café

Published and compiled by Orion House

Copyright © 2023 by Daliah Barkan. All rights reserved.

Cover Design by Vincenzo Vigliarolo

ISBN 978-1-7392094-0-7

Printed by Parbpim Co. Ltd, Nonthaburi, Thailand. First edition, June 2023.

www.orionhealing.com
orionhealing@gmail.com

License Notes:

This book is licensed for your personal enjoyment only. Please consult with an educated, informed healthcare practitioner or naturopath for health information.
No part of this publication may be reproduced, or transmitted in any form or by any means, electronic, mechanical, photocopying or otherwise, without written permission of the publisher, except in the case of brief quotation with reference to the title or author.

Special discounts and healing services are available through Orion, please contact our Thailand retreat center to explore ideas and opportunities.

Cooking is love made visible

Orion is a spiritual home for so many and, like in all good homes, our food is testimony to love. This book is dedicated to my husband, Ari Barkan, whose vision has alchemised the lives of many people, and to my children who inspire me to create a better future for us all.

I am grateful to see this dream to its fruition. To my parents, who gave me the foundation, love and support from which to rise; to my two aunties who taught me the magic and medicine within the plants, you know who you are ~ I thank you both.

To Ziv Ben Tzvi, our partner in Orion, thank you for your support, friendship and most of all your trust. Love and gratitude to all those who come to our Healing Centre, and those who supported us from small beginnings in 2005, before the North-West Side of Koh Phangan was on the trail. Thank you also to all our extended Orion family, teachers and facilitators, and everyone who contributed to this book and inspired our recipes from their vast health knowledge. Thank you Sussana Tose, who made the idea of this book more tangible, and to Rebecca Haas, whose help with coordination early on was priceless.

Great appreciation to Hila Gersztenkorn for her artistry, unique design talent and patience, and huge thanks to Vincenzo Vigliarolo for his expert graphic design skill set, which sealed the project. Massive thanks to Colleen Thornton, who found the exact words to bring the recipes alive on paper. I remember reading her description of *Om Ramen* and I knew she was the one!

Thanks to Brian Gruber for being a 'literary Uncle' to me. Thank you to Jade Richardson, my editor, for your time, dedication and expertise. Thanks to all our staff, especially our kitchen team, most of whom are political refugees from Burma and living far from their families. May peace prevail in your land.

To Bryce Draper who is featured in this book.
Fly high our dear friend, may we be reunited again.

With Love,

Let food be thy medicine and medicine be thy food

Hippocrates

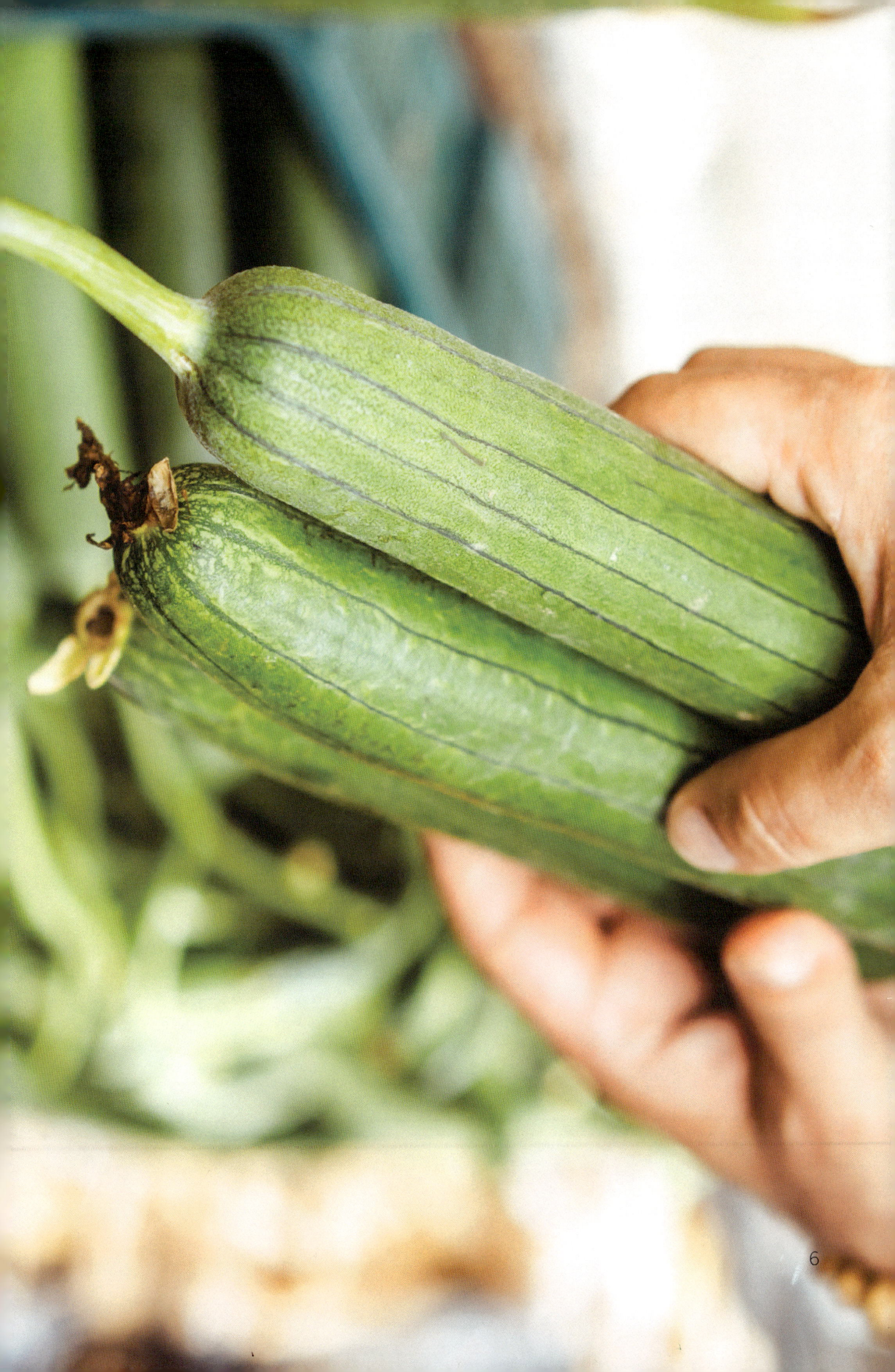

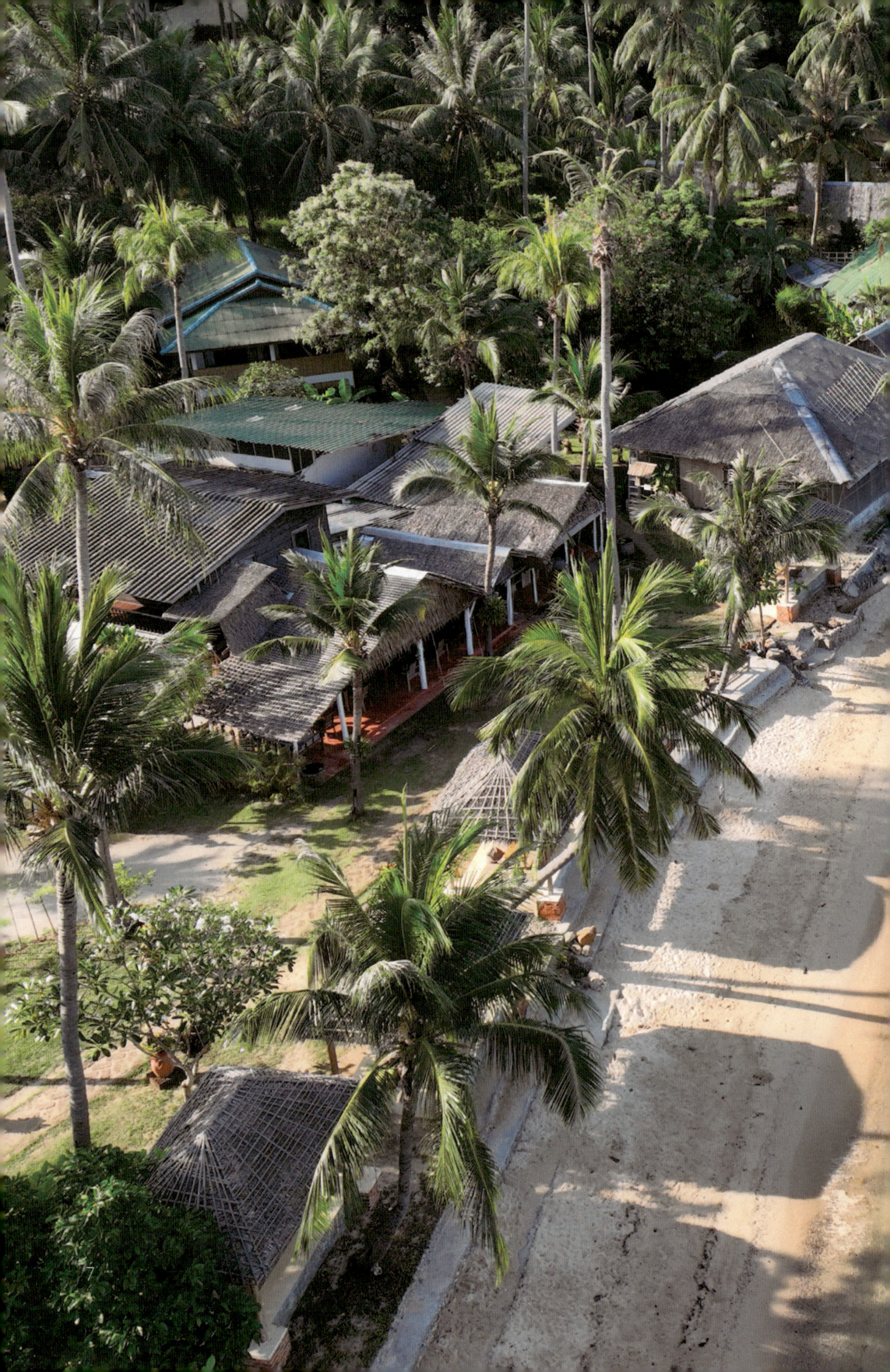

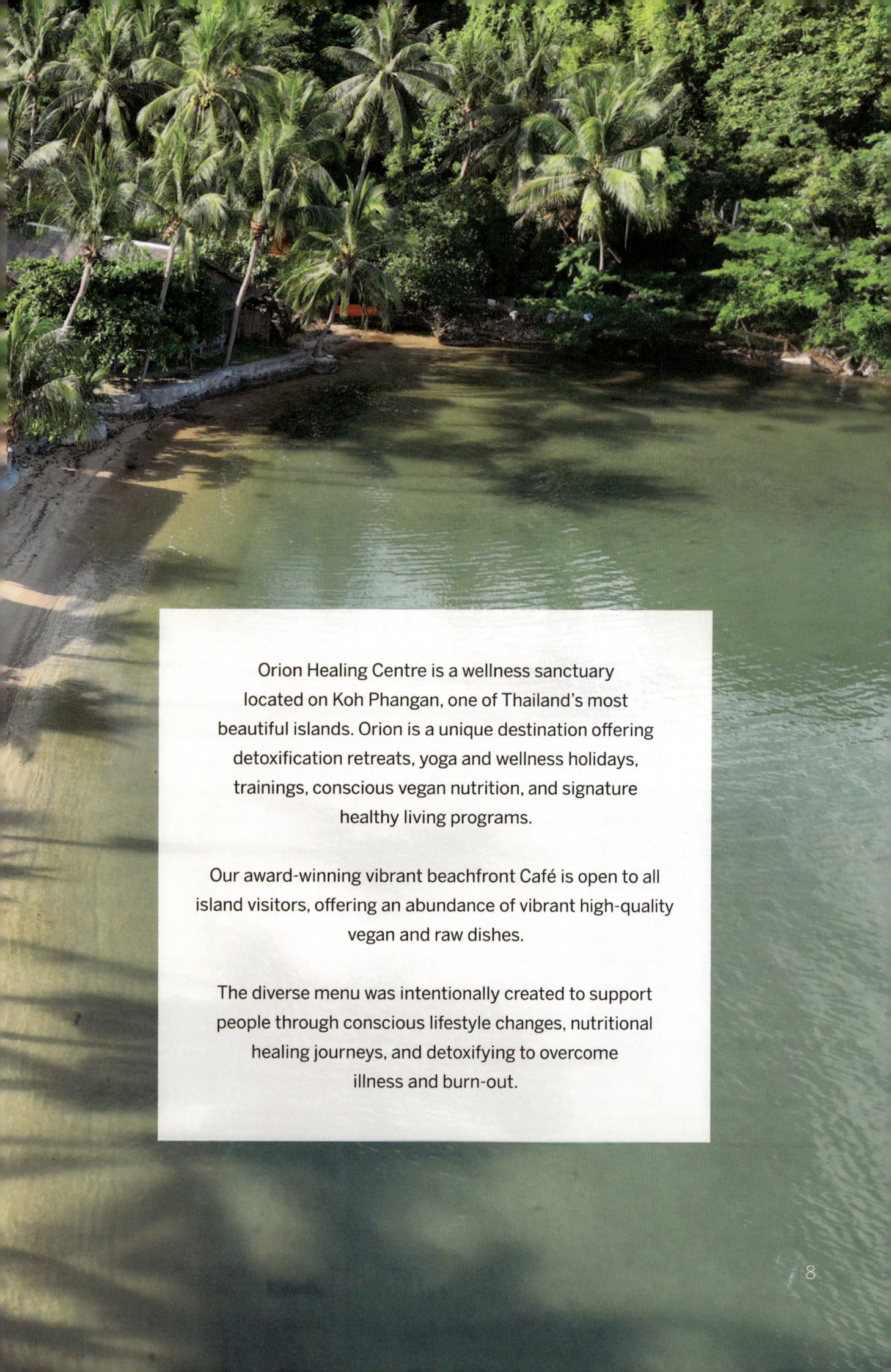

Orion Healing Centre is a wellness sanctuary located on Koh Phangan, one of Thailand's most beautiful islands. Orion is a unique destination offering detoxification retreats, yoga and wellness holidays, trainings, conscious vegan nutrition, and signature healthy living programs.

Our award-winning vibrant beachfront Café is open to all island visitors, offering an abundance of vibrant high-quality vegan and raw dishes.

The diverse menu was intentionally created to support people through conscious lifestyle changes, nutritional healing journeys, and detoxifying to overcome illness and burn-out.

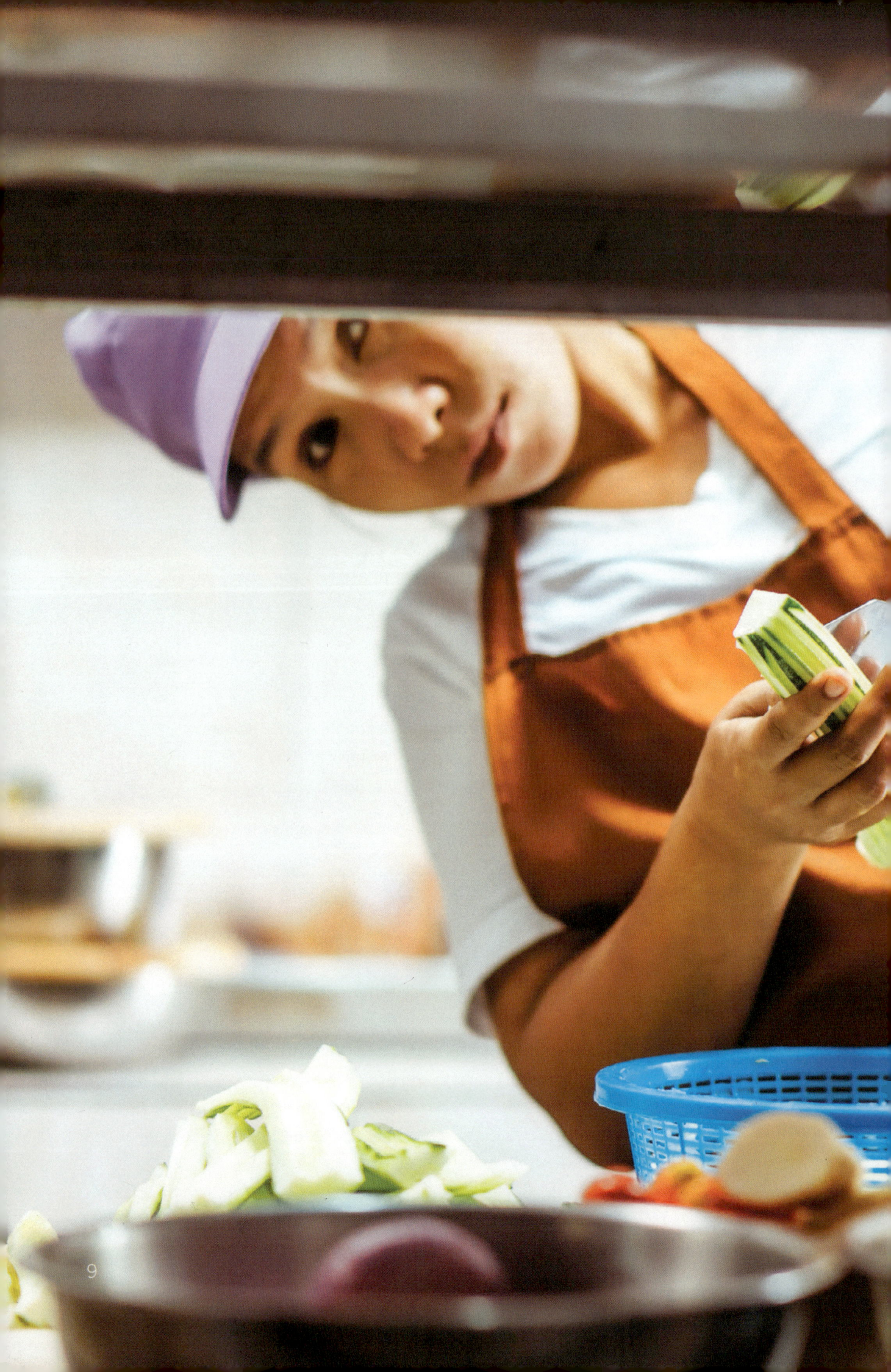

The food at Orion is lovingly created by our restaurant team.
Ingredients come from all around the world: quinoa from Peru,
cacao from Bali, and tahini from the Middle East.

We source most of our fruits and vegetables locally from the region ~
from hydroponic farms, we gather herbs, edible flowers, sprouted seeds
and fruits. We collect produce from local fresh markets, as well as from
our own land, where we grow sunflower sprouts,
wheatgrass and papaya.

We selected the best of our extensive plant-based Orion Café menu for
this book. Our intention is to continue to nourish you with vibrant food
and fresh beverages even after your stay on the island is over.
You'll enjoy healthy and delicious raw dishes, succulent salads, smoothies,
and juices that help balance your body's pH and increase your vitality,
radiance and energy.

Food of the highest vibration elevates body, mind and spirit.
Through a conscious and effective diet we can improve our overall
health, immunity and wellbeing.

Our mission is to create an organic movement
of change through lifestyle and food choices.

Thank you for joining us.

Table of contents

DRINKS
Almond Milk — 15
Chia Lemonade — 17

FRESH JUICES
Go Green — 21
Immunity — 23
Pink Punch — 25

SMOOTHIES
Goodbye Fun-Guy — 29
Golden Milk — 31
Ari's Breakfast — 33
Solar Plexus — 35
Hanuman — 37
Omega — 39

ELIXIRS
Alkalizer — 43
Wellness Shot — 45
Apple Snap — 47

BREAKFAST
Orion Super Papaya — 51
Chia Bomb — 53
Yogi Breakfast — 55
Green Smoothie Bowl — 57
Vegan Omelette — 59

SALADS
Thai Papaya Salad — 63
Rainbow Quinoa Salad — 65
Caesar Salad — 67

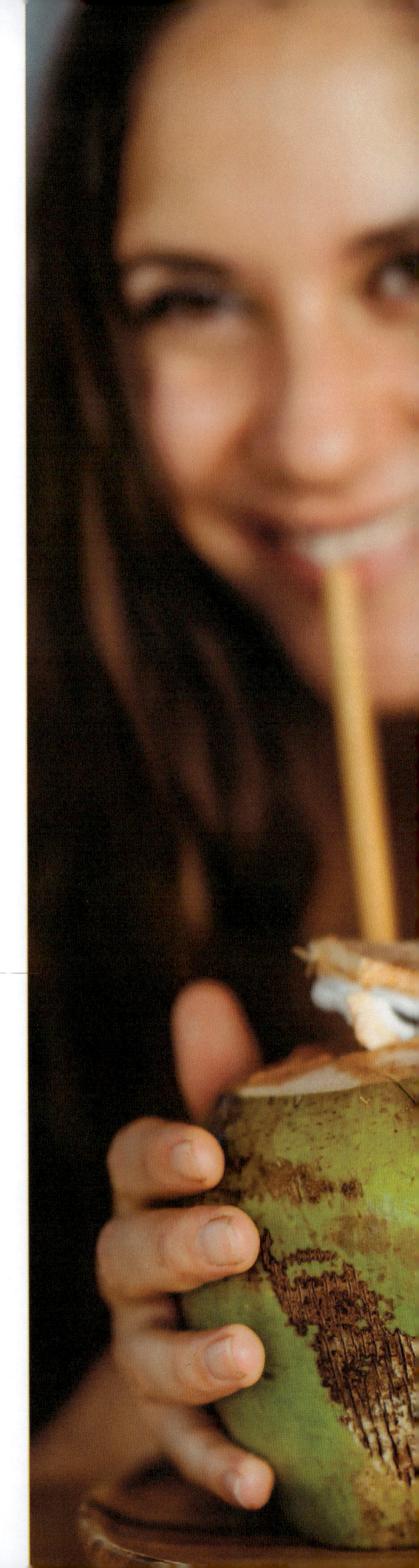

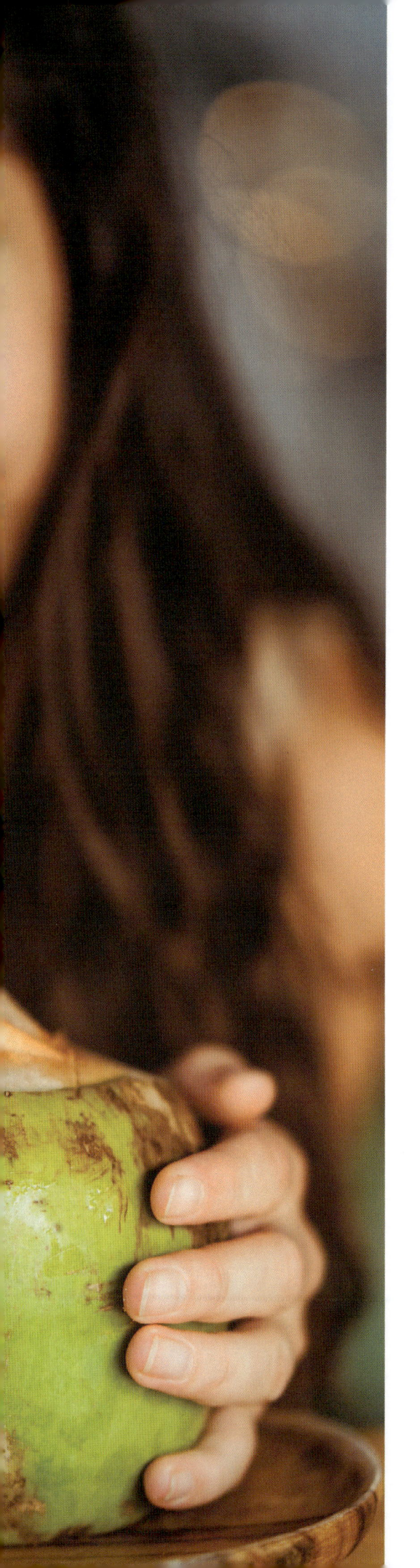

RAW FOOD

Raw Trinity Tacos	71
Raw Rainbow Sushi	73
Zucchini Friendships	75
Raw Cauliflower Rice	77
Cucumber & Spirulina Soup	79
Raw Gazpacho	81

MAIN DISHES

Bliss Bowl	85
Beetroot Burger	87
Om Ramen	89
Dhal Tadka	91
Coconut Curry	93
Spicy Meaty Mushrooms	95

DESSERTS

Raw Cheesecake	99
Raw Chocolate Fudge	101
Raw Snickers Bar	103
Mint Cupcake	105

SAUCES & SIDES

Orange Olive Oil Dressing	109
Tomato Salsa	110
Raw Seeded Crackers	111
Baba Ganoush	113
Sweet Potato Fries	115
Roasted Chickpeas	117
Soy Sesame Dressing	118
Ginger Lemon Tahini	119
Mango & Kaffir Lime	121
Kale Pesto	123
Roasty Tomatoes	124
Tomato Ketchup	125
Cashew Cheese	127
Purple Sauerkraut	129
Vegan Parmesan	131
Caesar Basil Pesto	132
Caesar Dressing	133
Coconut Bacon	134

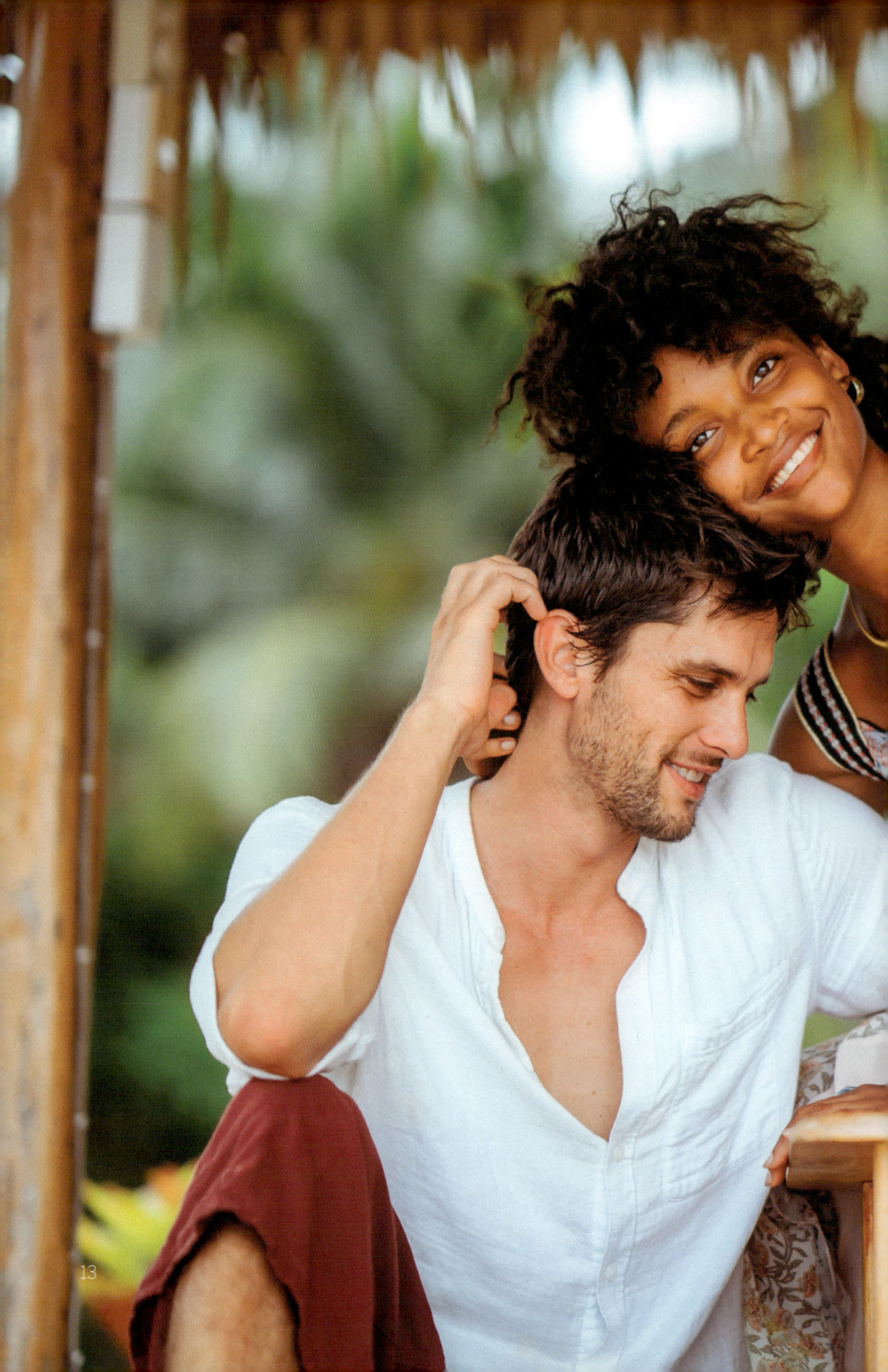

Drinks

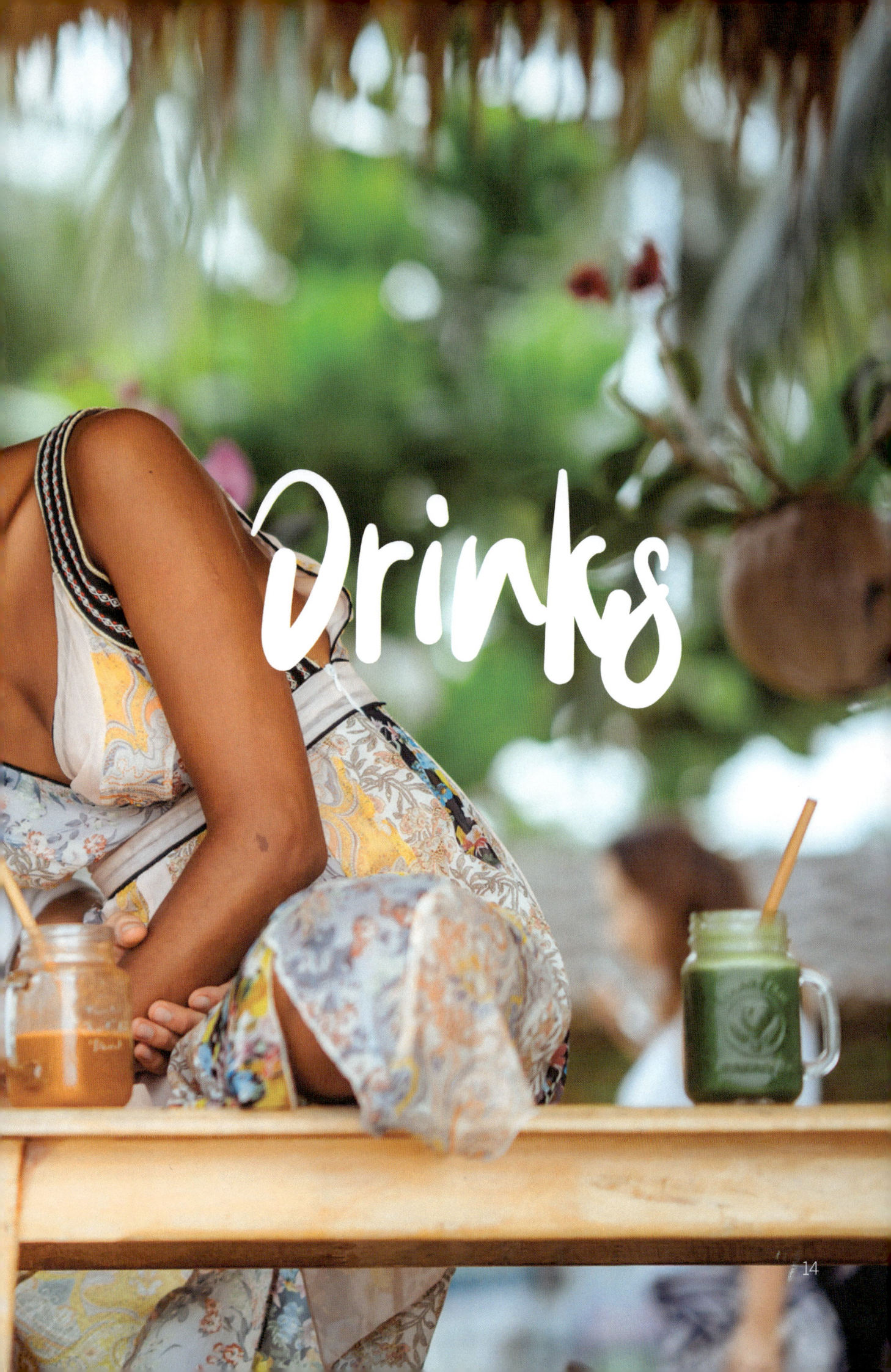

Almond Milk

Luscious and light, almond milk has a velvety texture and nutty flavour that enhances smoothie bowls, puddings, and makes the very best vegan mayo. Soaking the almonds releases their abundant nutrients. Enjoy this low-cal milk alternative hot or chilled, and go nuts with ideas for the pulpy extras.

INGREDIENTS

1 cup Almonds
(soaked in water for 10 - 12 hours)

4 cups Water

Ice, if desired

INSTRUCTIONS

Drain the soaked almonds and rinse them well. In a blender, combine almonds with fresh water, and blend until the milk looks creamy. Strain through a mesh nut milk bag, squeezing out the extra almond milk and store in an airtight container in the fridge for up to 4 days.

Serving Size: 4 cups
Preparation Time: 10 minutes

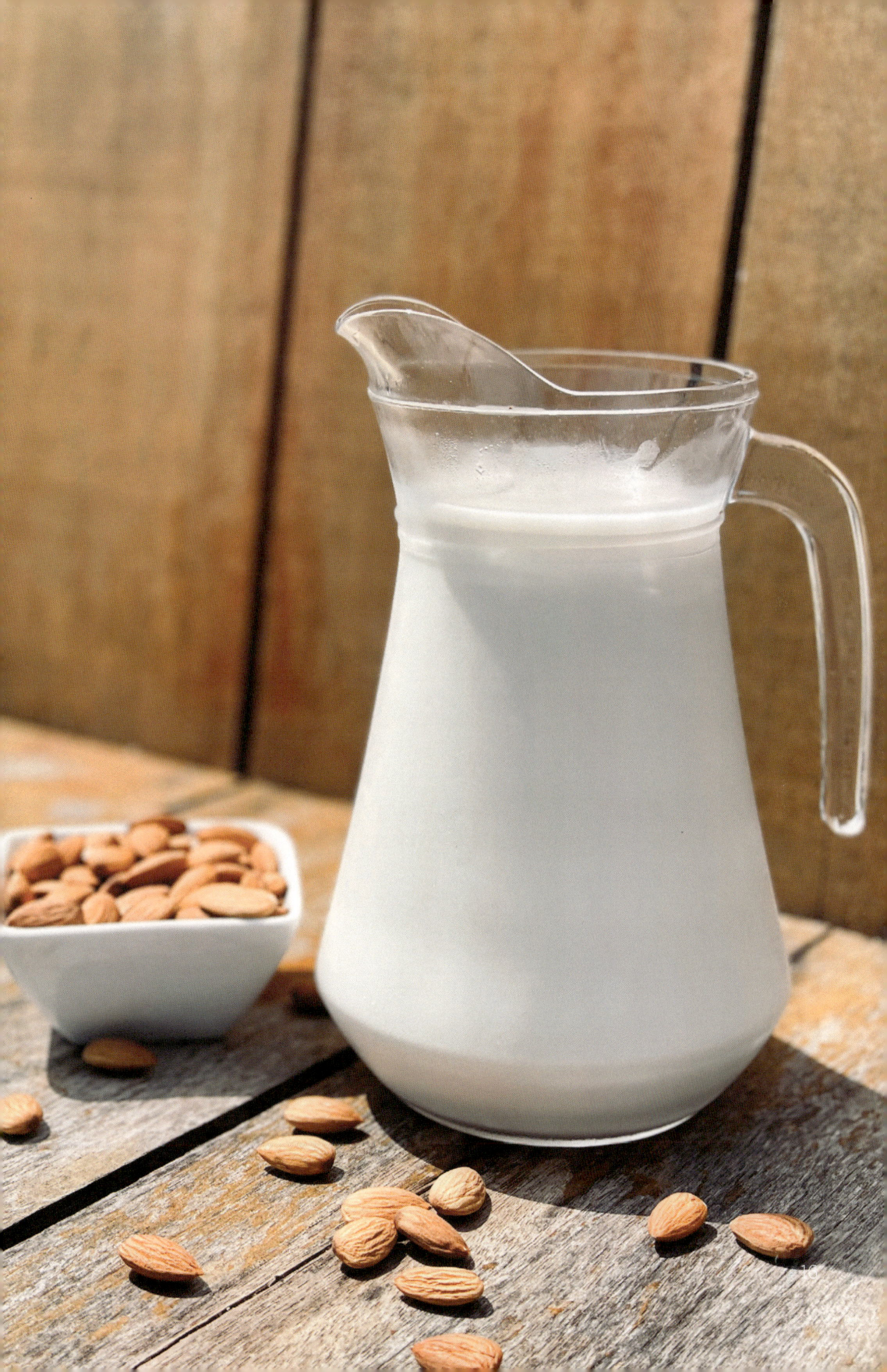

Delightfully tart without overwhelm; citrus-drunk chia seeds decorate this most pleasing childhood favourite. Hand-squeezed lemon, coconut nectar, and fragrant mint leaves meet fresh water and slippery chia seeds in a fusion of refreshing, thirst-quenching love. Tastes like long summer days and washes down like jungle rain.

INGREDIENTS

1 tbsp Chia seeds

3 tbsp Coconut syrup

3 tbsp Lemon juice

7 – 8 Mint leaves

1½ cups Cold water

Ice, if desired

INSTRUCTIONS

Mix the lemon juice, coconut syrup, and water in a glass jar. Then, add the chia seeds and mint leaves, and place in the fridge for 15 minutes. The chia seeds will absorb some of the water and plump up.

Serving Size: 1
Preparation Time: 25 minutes

Coconut syrup is a healthy and natural alternative to sugar and is high in enzymes and minerals. Coconut trees often grow in rich volcanic soils where the roots are able to draw an abundance of nutrients up from the ground. The consistency and colour of coconut syrup is like maple syrup, yet the taste is deep, rich and caramelly.

Chia Lemonade

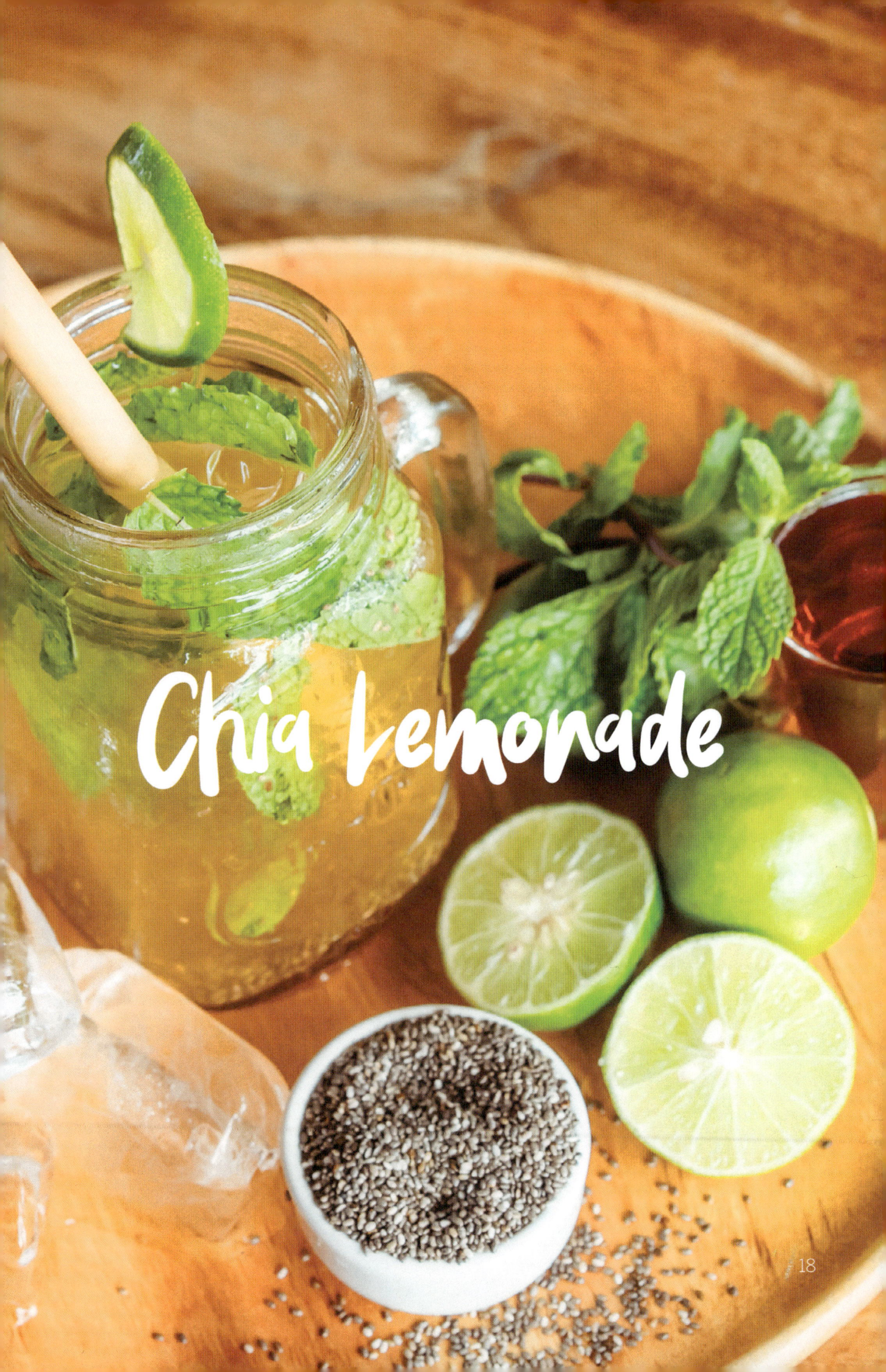

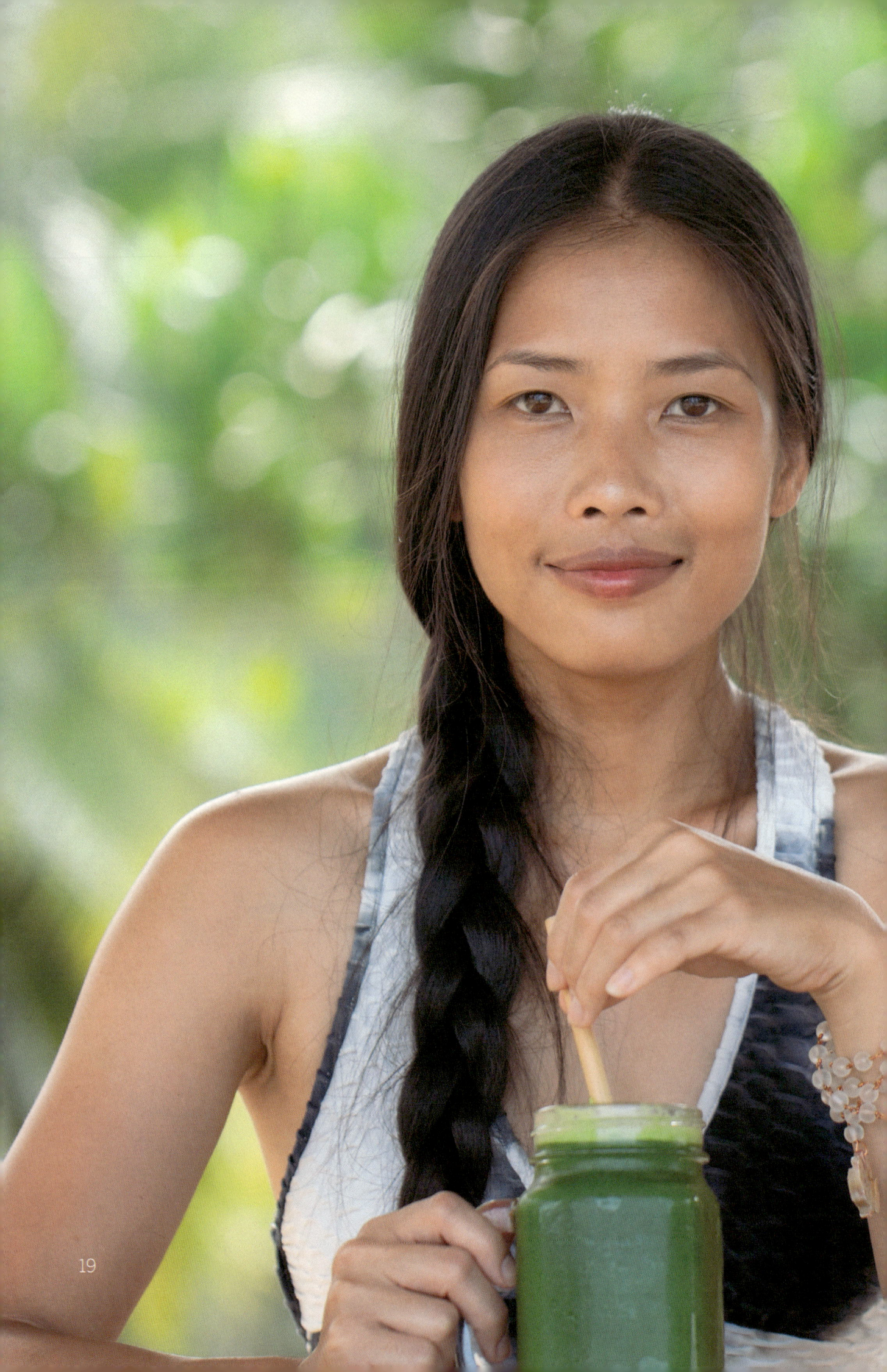

Juices

Go Green

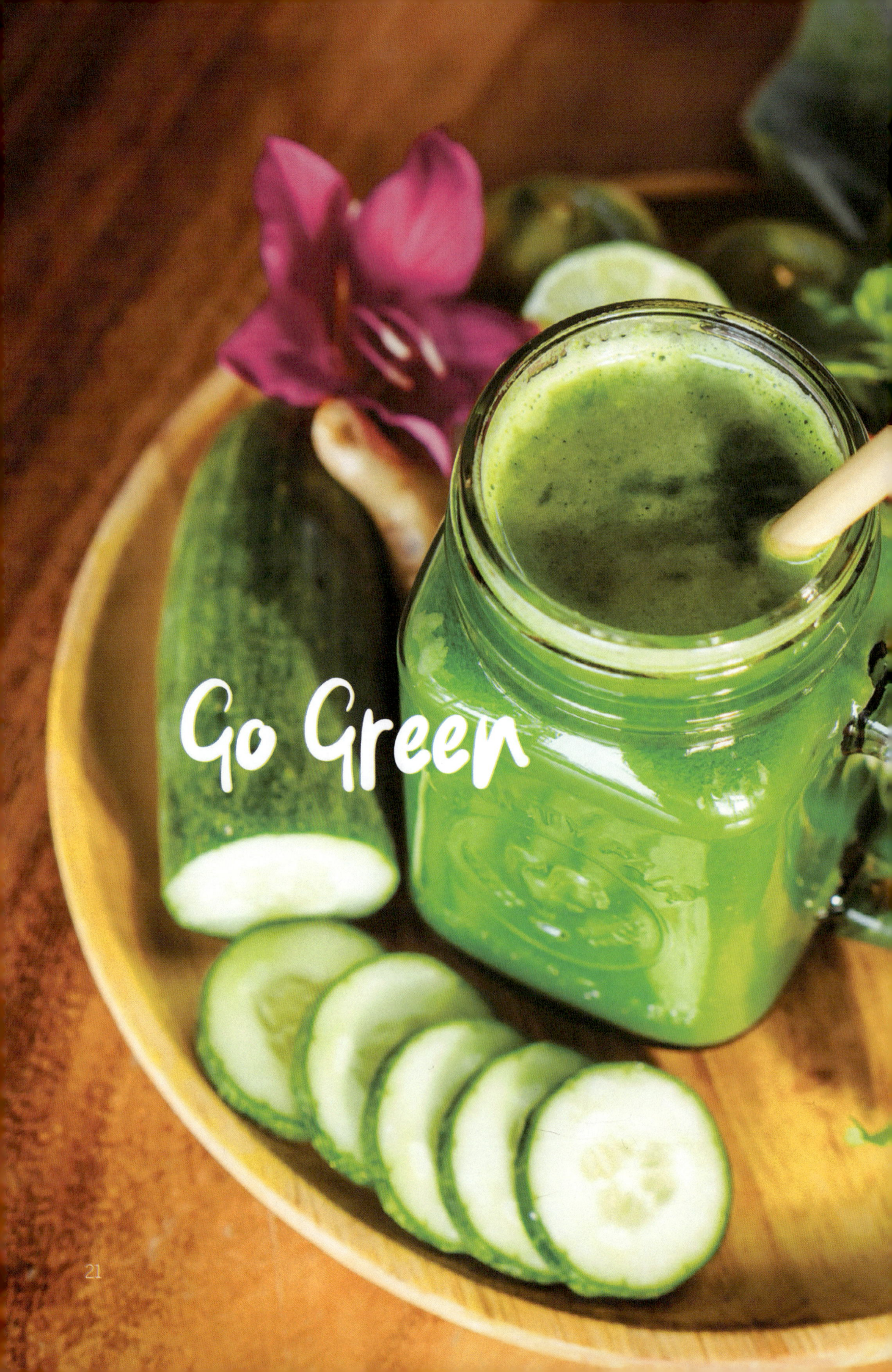

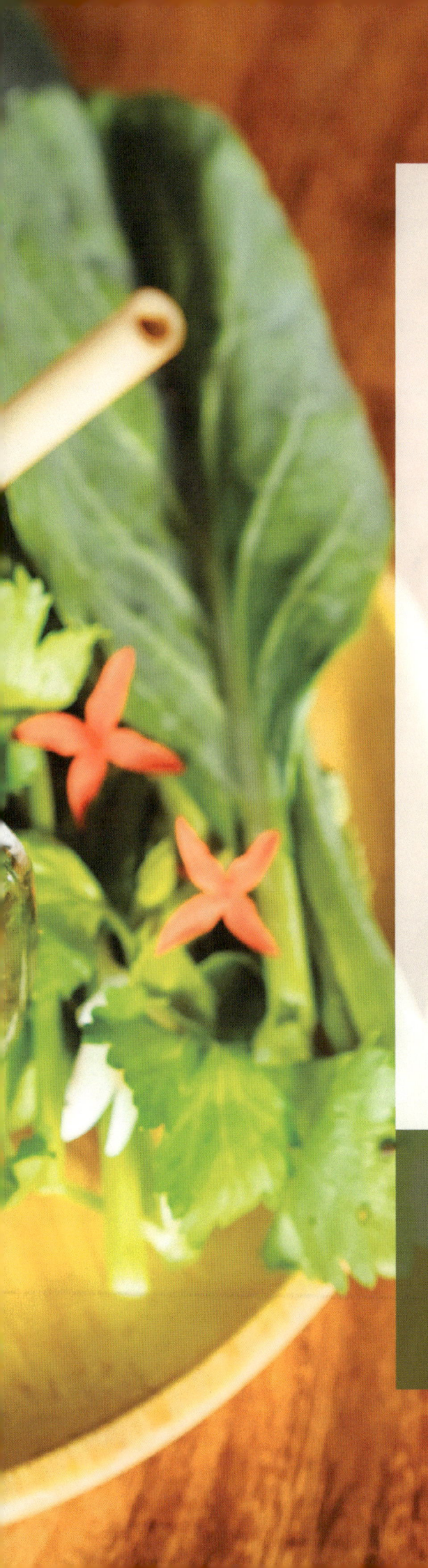

Fresh and rewarding with a brave kick of ginger. For the love of kale and the entire green veg kingdom, devote your heart health to this super cleanser. Cucumber and celery hydrate thirsty cells and flush out fatigue. Mineral-rich kale boosts Vitamin C levels, and ginger prepares the palate. A sneaky squeeze of lime tops off this green tango.

INGREDIENTS

350 gr Cucumber

40 gr Celery leaf

100 gr Kale leaf

10 gr Ginger

Juice from ½ Lime

INSTRUCTIONS

Feed each ingredient, one by one, into a slow cold-press juicer.

Serving Size: 1
Preparation Time: 5 minutes

There are many different types of kale. The leaves are green or purple, and have either a smooth or curly shape. Kale is extremely high in Vitamin C and other important antioxidants. A single cup of raw kale contains more Vitamin C than an orange!

Spirited, blood-balancing, and sensational; orange and carrot have always belonged together. Here, celery makes a majestic entrance. The flavour dynamic of this energising earthy juice both lifts and grounds. Drink your way to equanimity.

INGREDIENTS

250 gr Orange

250 gr Carrot

30 gr Celery

Ice, if desired

INSTRUCTIONS

Feed each ingredient, one by one, into a slow cold-press juicer.

Serving Size: 1
Preparation Time: 5 minutes

Celery is surprisingly dense with vitamins and minerals, despite its high water content. It has a low glycemic index, so it won't spike blood sugar no matter how much you consume, and it helps fight inflammation.

Immunity

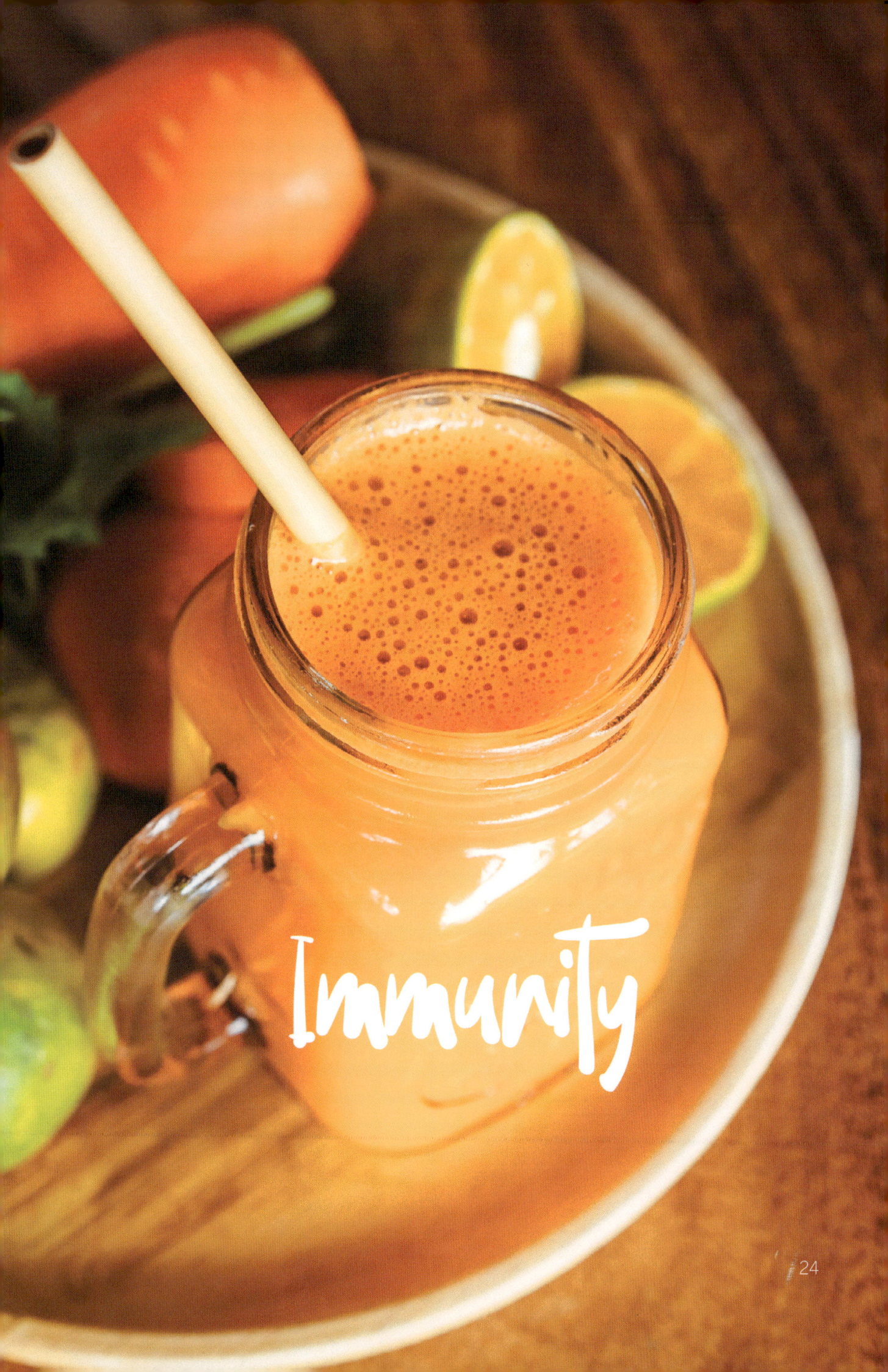

You might wonder if the Brahmans created this other-worldly nectar. Sweet n' earthy, blood-boosting beetroot conquers the colour mix, but vibrant pineapple, with its fibrous flesh, kicks up the sweetness score. Ginger's robust heat lends a surge of strength and warms the throat. Loving, punchy, and full of flair.

INGREDIENTS

300 gr Pineapple

100 gr Beetroot

10 gr Ginger

INSTRUCTIONS

Feed each ingredient, one by one, into a slow cold-press juicer.

Serving Size: 1
Preparation Time: 5 minutes

Beetroot contains betalains, the pigment that gives beets their incandescent red tint. They're why beets are a prime candidate for producing natural dyes, especially when boiled. The roots themselves are loaded with micronutrients that offer several health benefits.

Pink Punch

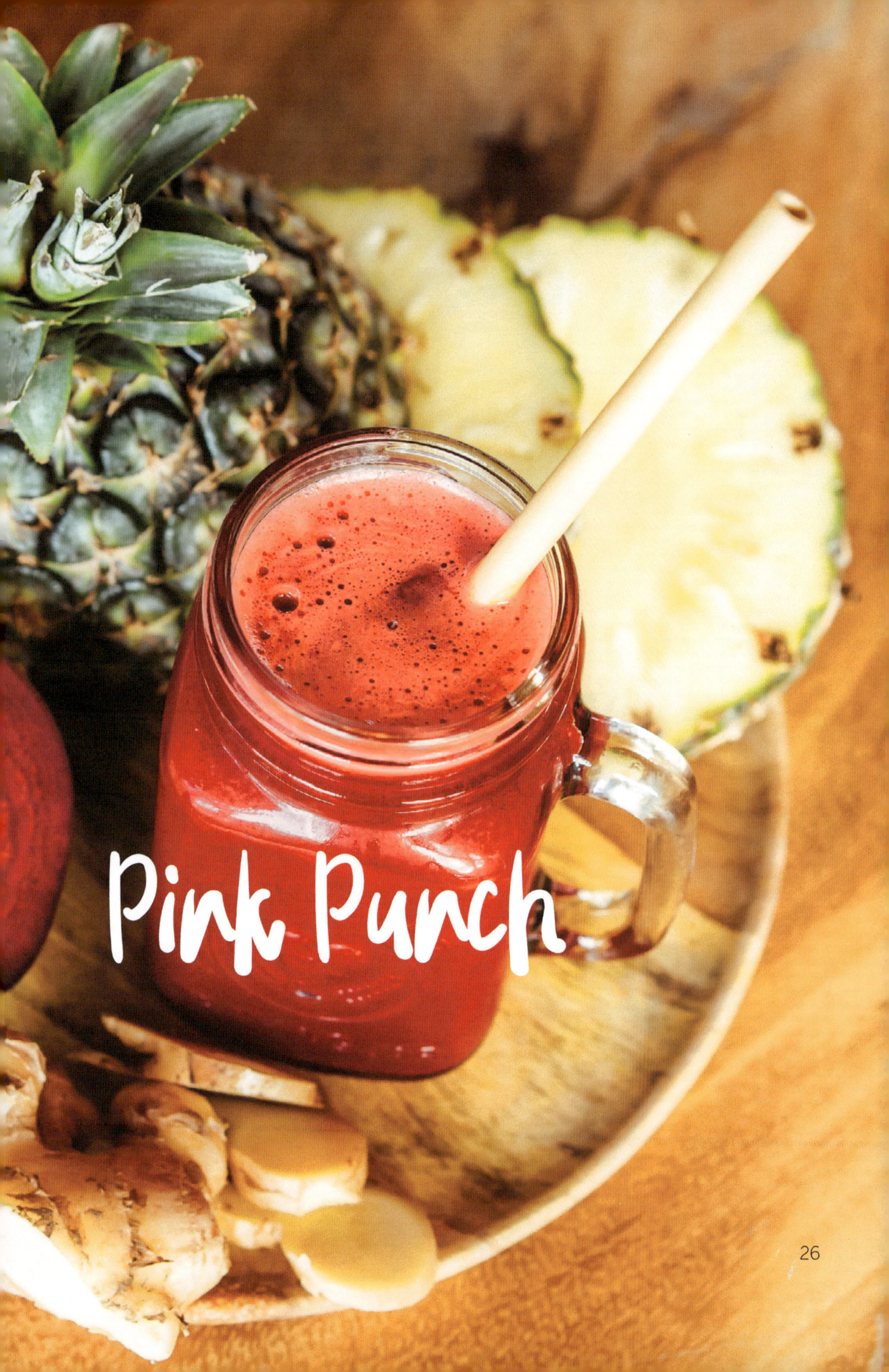

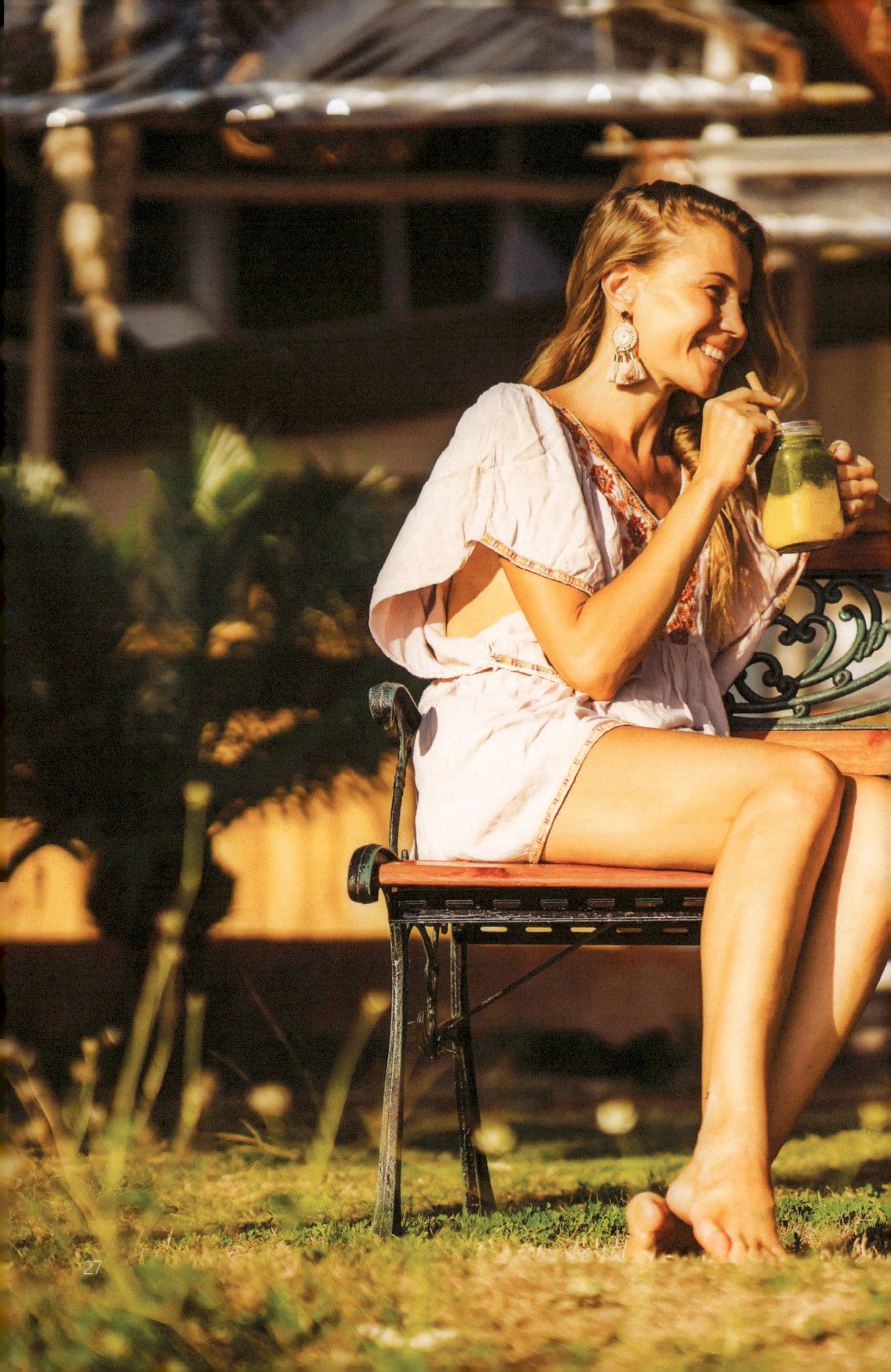

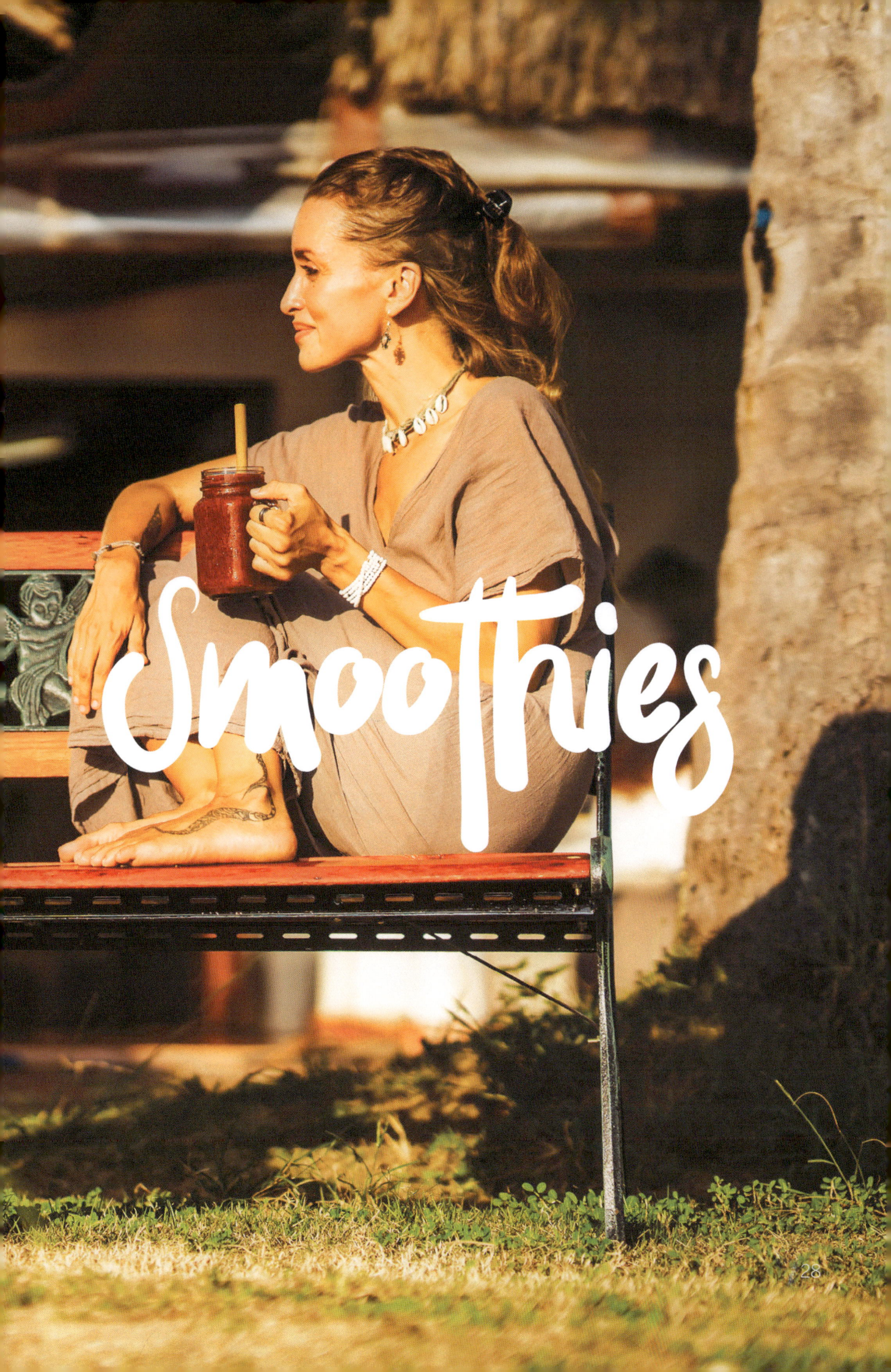

Smoothies

Goodbye Fun-Guy

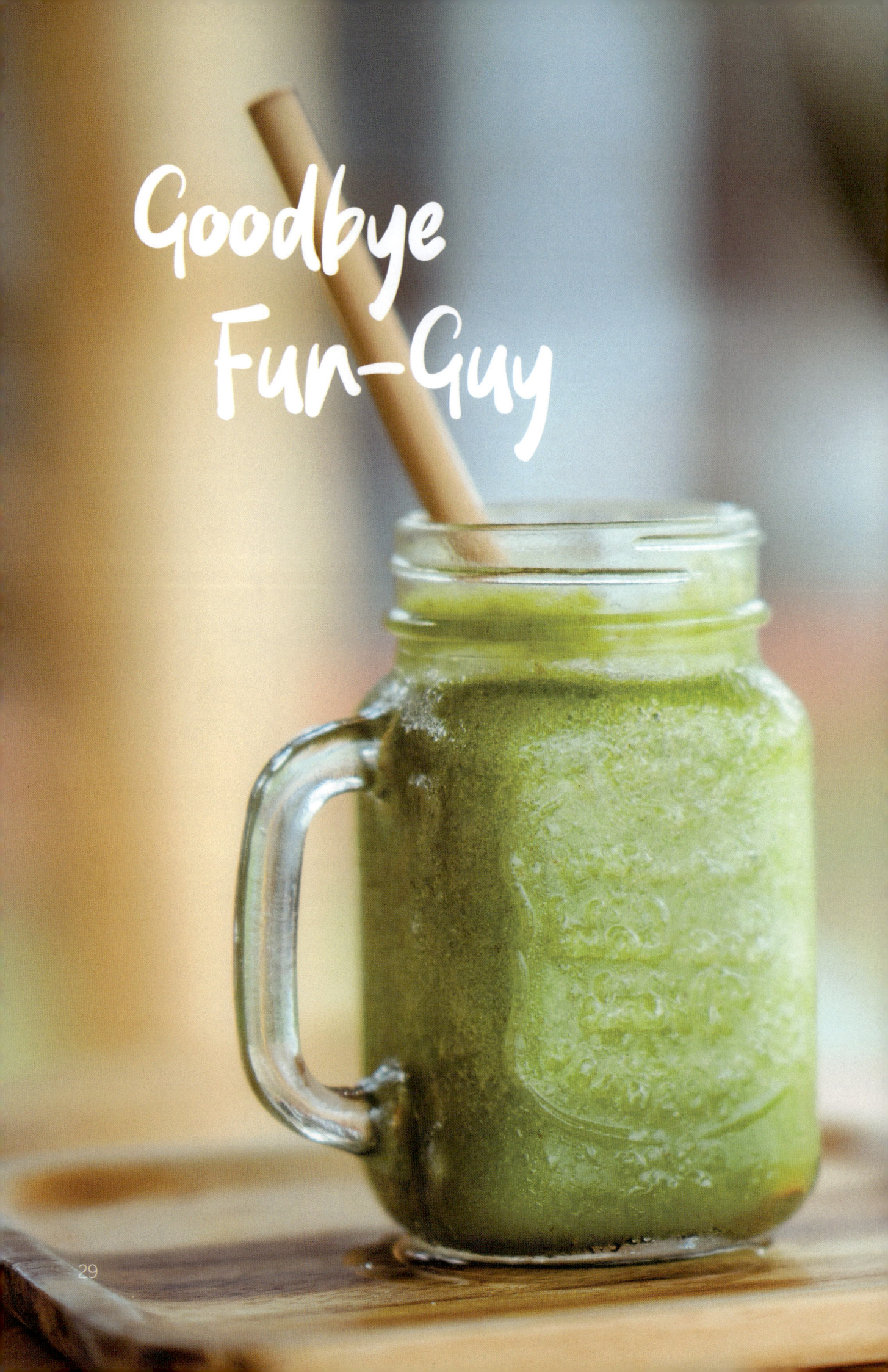

A perfect potion for cleansing your spirit and giving candida the boot. Raw leafy kale meets sweet pineapple and a hearty kick of ginger in this fresh n' frothy smoothie, kissed with warm, delicate cinnamon. Coconut oil makes it a warrior in the face of unwanted fungi.

INGREDIENTS

100 gr Kale leaf

200 gr Pineapple

5 gr Ginger

1 tbsp Coconut oil

1 tsp Cinnamon powder

4 – 5 Ice cubes

INSTRUCTIONS

Mix all ingredients together in a high-speed blender.

Serving Size: 1
Preparation Time: 5 minutes

Cinnamon is one of our favourite spices for its amazing health benefits. It gives juices, shakes, and smoothies a beautiful taste and is one of the most delicious and healthy spices on the planet.

Gloriously creamy, this coconut milkshake might be your #1 way to reap all the benefits of turmeric. A luscious concoction chock-full of curcuminoids; inflammation-fighting compounds that give turmeric root its regal orange tint. Frozen banana adds a chill factor.

INGREDIENTS

200 gr Frozen banana

1 tbsp Turmeric juice

10 gr Ginger

¼ cup Coconut milk

INSTRUCTIONS

Mix all ingredients together in a high-speed blender.

Serving Size: 1
Preparation Time: 5 minutes

For thousands of years, Ayurvedic practitioners have sung the praises of this miraculous golden root, most commonly known for its anti-inflammatory properties, especially when combined with black pepper. Turmeric gives curries their bold orange hue. When consumed as a fresh-pressed juice or smoothie, it will wow your senses back to the present.

Golden Milk

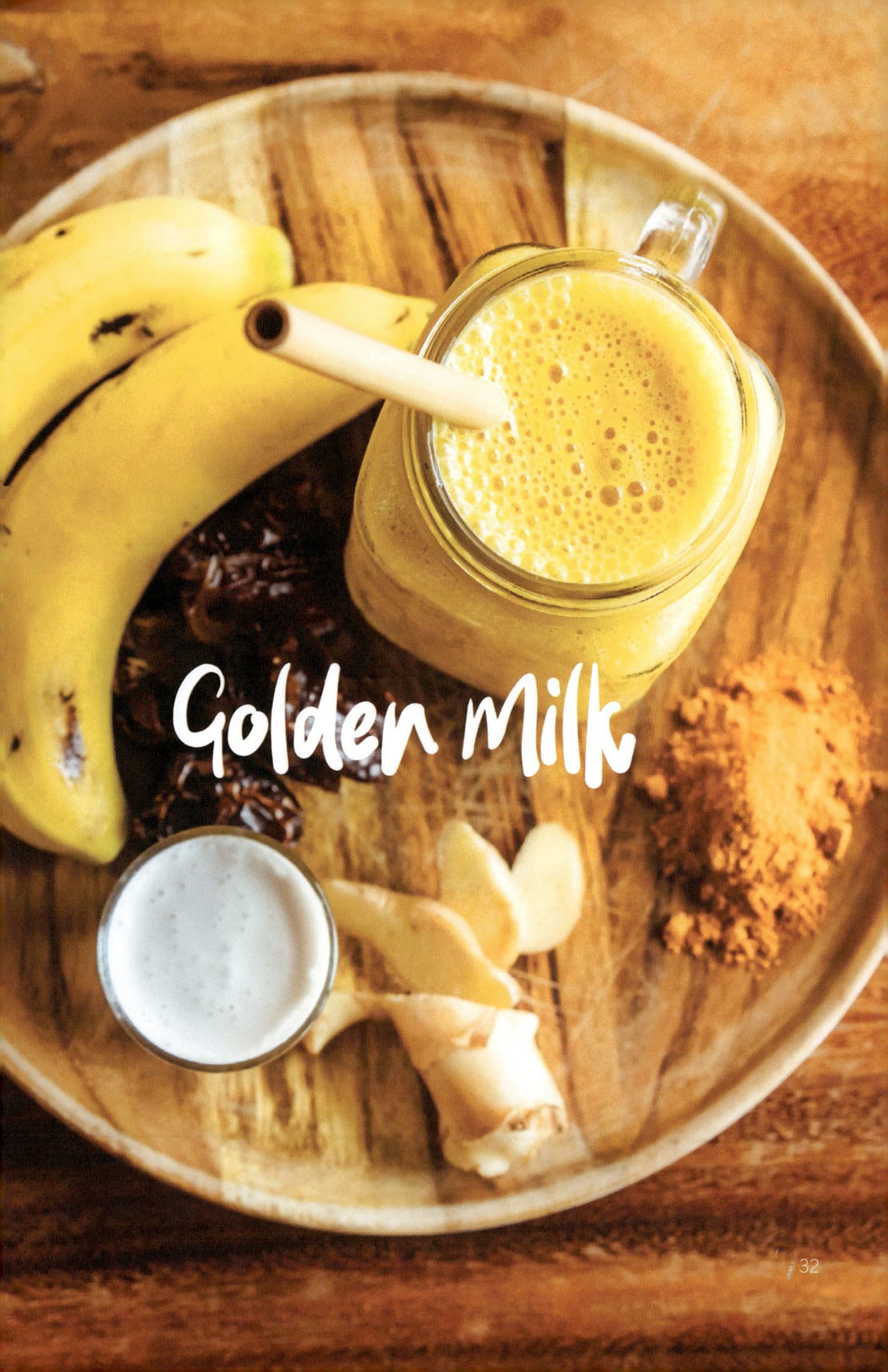

Ari's Breakfast

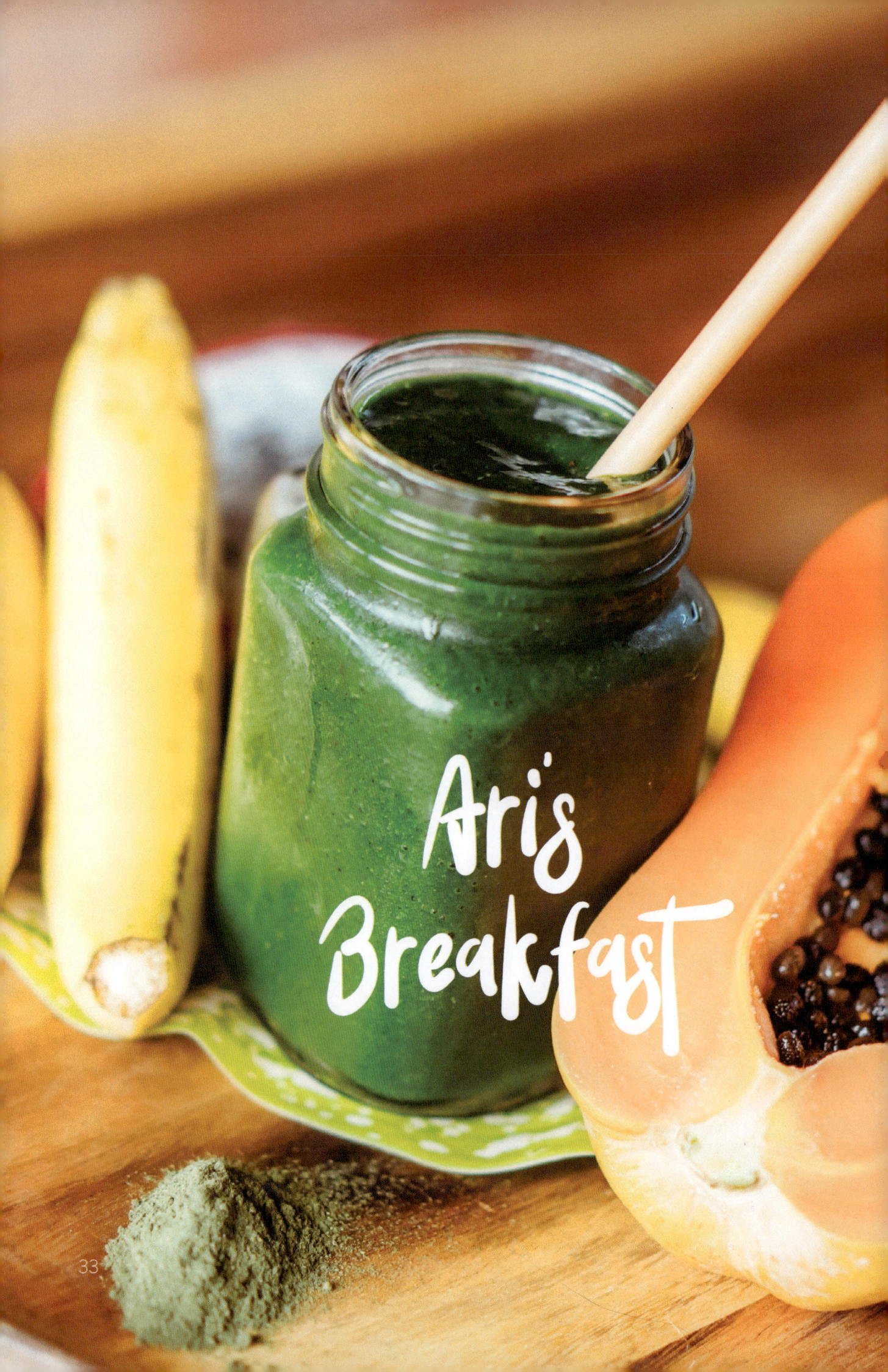

In a rush to get some solid sustenance in before you start your day? This fresh n' fruity smoothie will give you all the superpower you need. Inspired by Orion's co-founder and visionary, who digs his fruit bowl but doesn't always have the time to luxuriate over his breakfast.

INGREDIENTS

100 gr Mango

100 gr Banana

100 gr Papaya

100 gr Dragonfruit

1 tbsp Super green powder

INSTRUCTIONS

Mix all ingredients in a high-speed blender.

Serving Size: 1
Preparation Time: 5 minutes

Want to know what we put in our special blend of super green powder?
· Moringa powder · Chlorella powder · Spirulina powder
· Wheatgrass powder · Alfalfa powder

Meet your third and fourth chakras with this super-chill, layered and luscious taste bomb, and feel the expansion. Chlorella is a superb heart-opener, belly-buddy, and beneficial bacteria booster. Paired with sun-sugared mango and omega-rich chia seeds, this tropical tango is a commitment you'll dive into with pleasure.

INGREDIENTS

1ST LAYER

150 gr Frozen mango

½ cup Orange juice

1 tsp Chia seeds

2ND LAYER

150 gr Frozen mango

½ cup Orange juice

1 tsp Chia seeds

1 tbsp Chlorella powder

INSTRUCTIONS

Mix all ingredients for the first layer together in a high-speed blender. Pour the mixture into a large jar, to half of its capacity. Then mix the 2nd layer ingredients using a high-speed blender, and pour on top of the first layer.

Serving Size: 1
Preparation Time: 10 minutes

Chia seeds are nature's perfect food, delivering a massive amount of nutrients in very few calories. Antioxidants, fiber, protein, and omega-3 fatty acids give you a complete macro hit, plus lashings of micronutrients, including calcium and magnesium. To increase their bioavailability, soak for 20 minutes until they take on a soft, chewy texture.

Solar Plexus

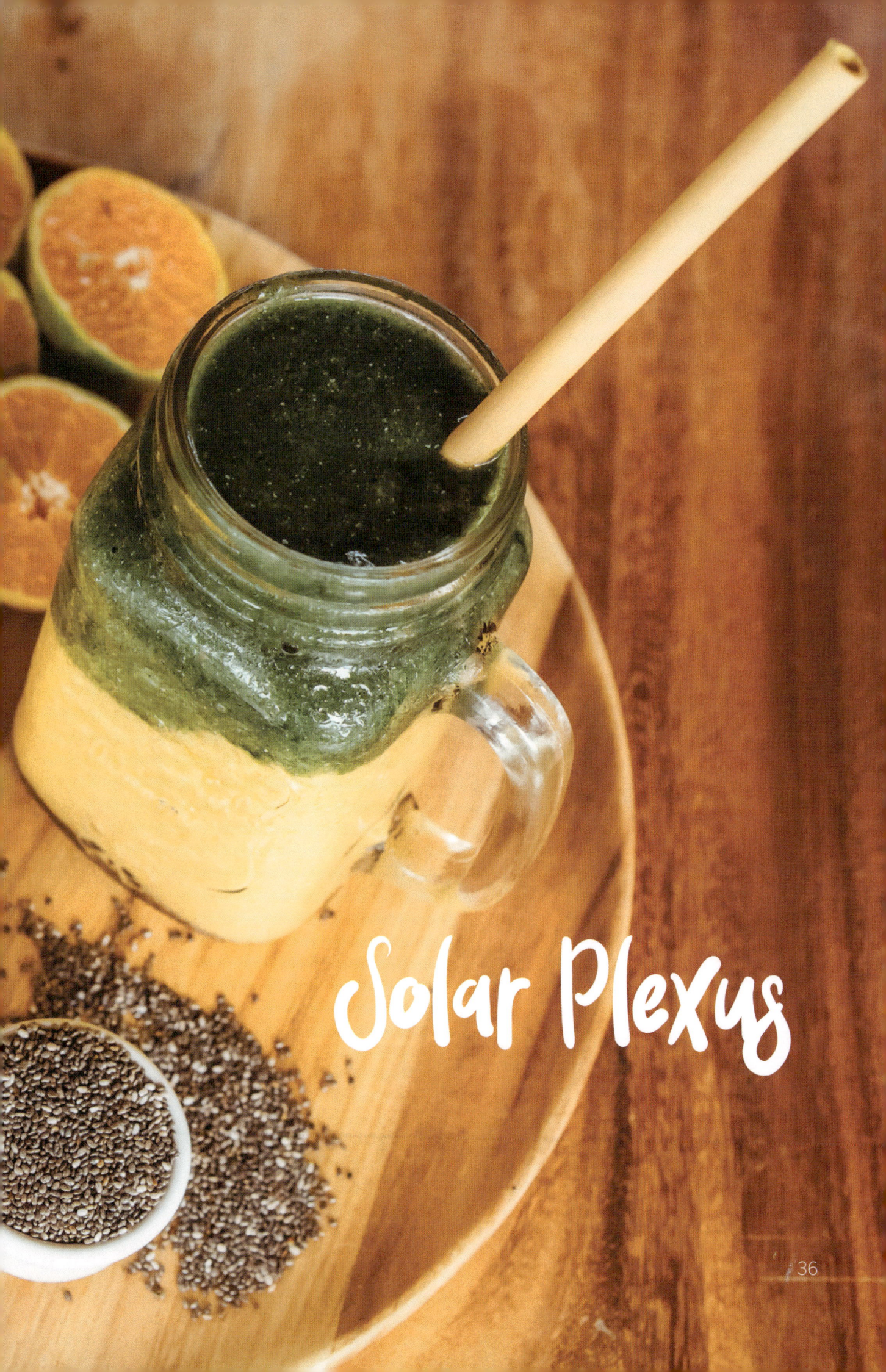

A symbol of strength and energy: Hanuman has soul. A decadent, creamy blend of the earth's food wonders: banana, coconut, chocolate, and dates power up the inner warrior with raw maca, a wild Peruvian ginseng root and aphrodisiac extraordinaire. Vanilla's natural sweetness lingers throughout.

INGREDIENTS

200 gr Frozen banana

100 gr Coconut meat

½ cup Coconut water

½ tbsp Maca powder

1 tbsp Raw cacao powder

2 Dates

1 tsp Vanilla essence

INSTRUCTIONS

Mix all ingredients together in a high-speed blender.

Serving Size: 1
Preparation Time: 5 minutes

Cacao powder is a gift of the Mayans, revered for its ability to lift the senses, boost the brain, and shine a light of love. The 'food of the Gods' is loaded with antioxidants that keep the childlike spirit alive.

Hanuman

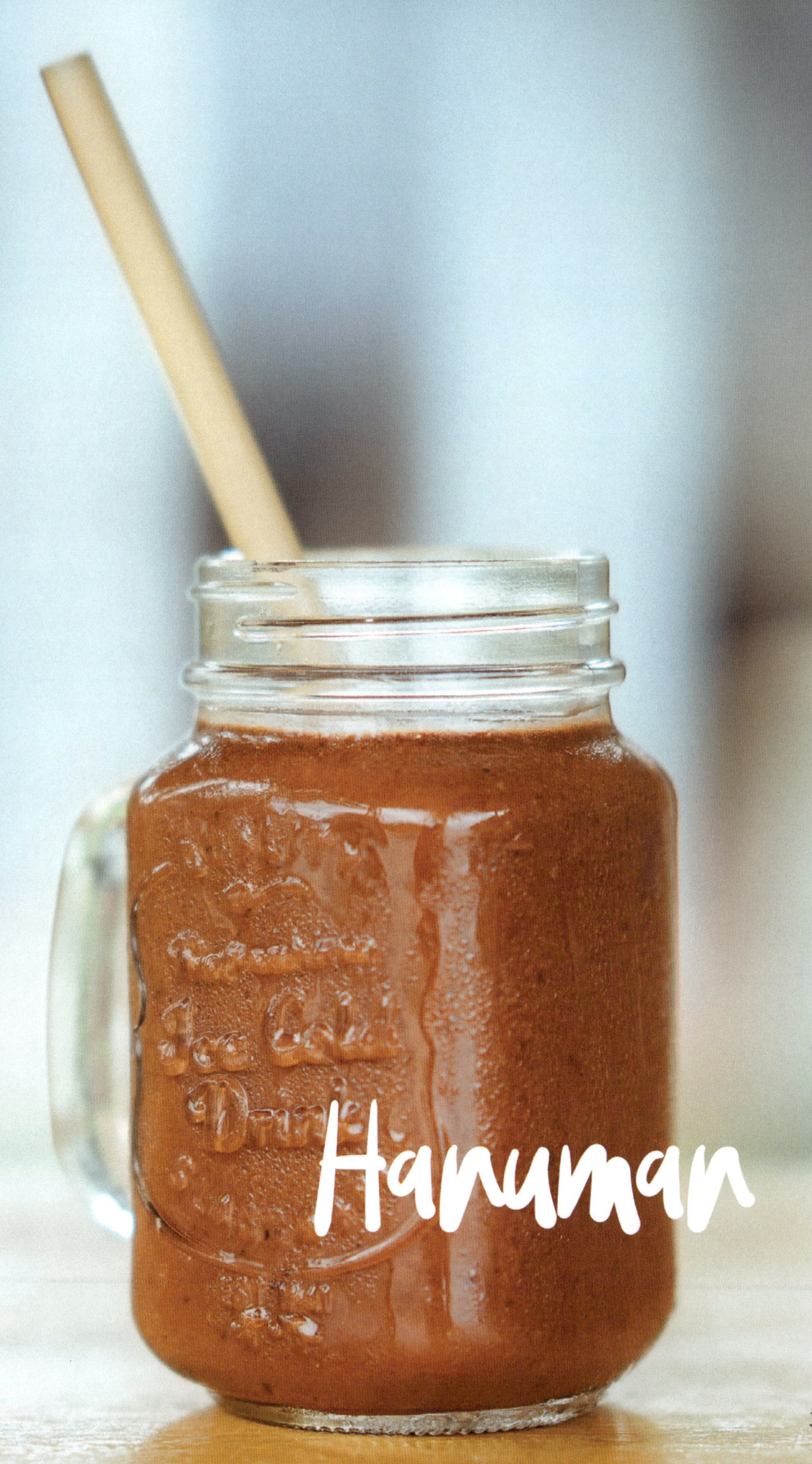

Omega

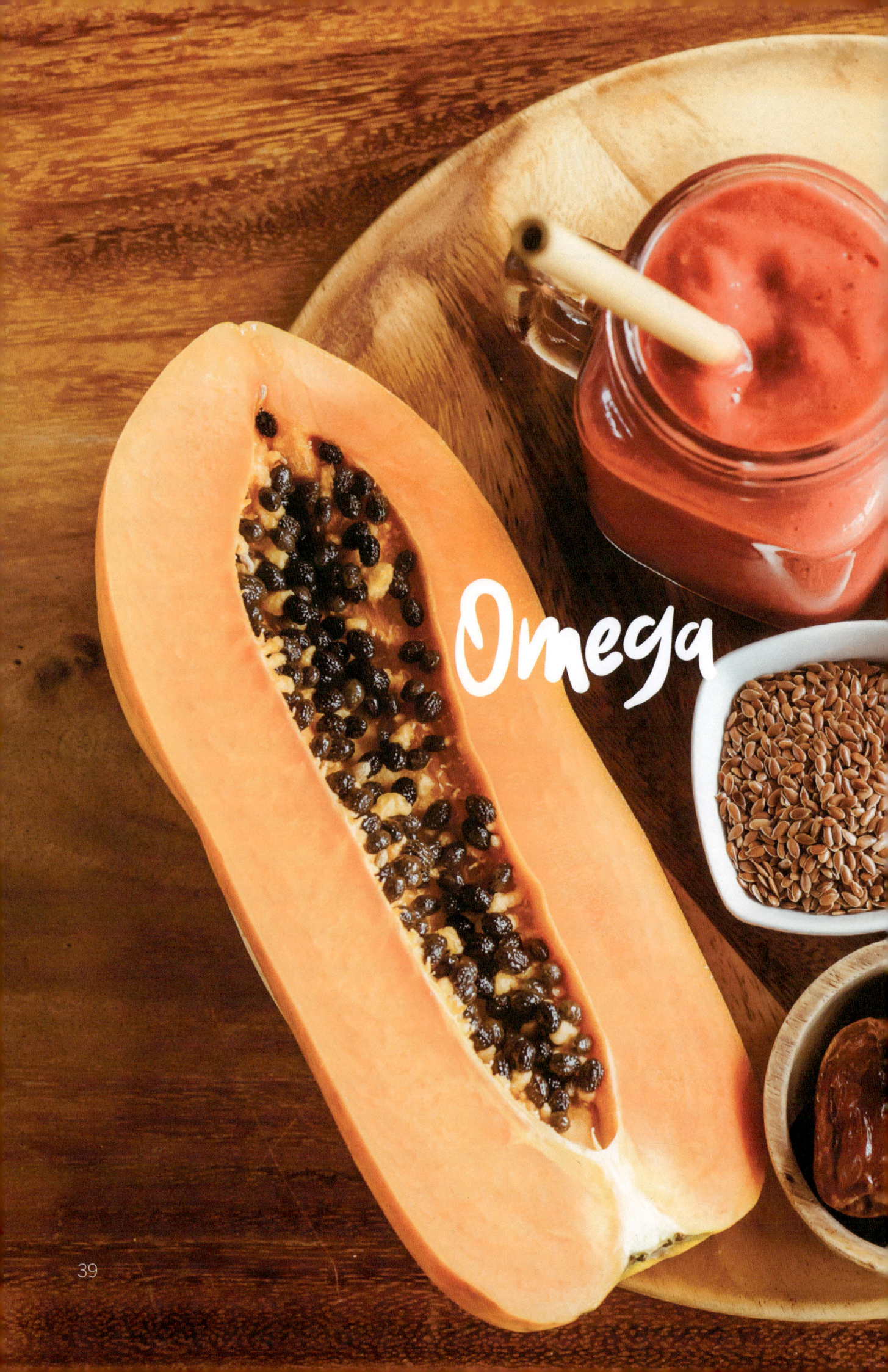

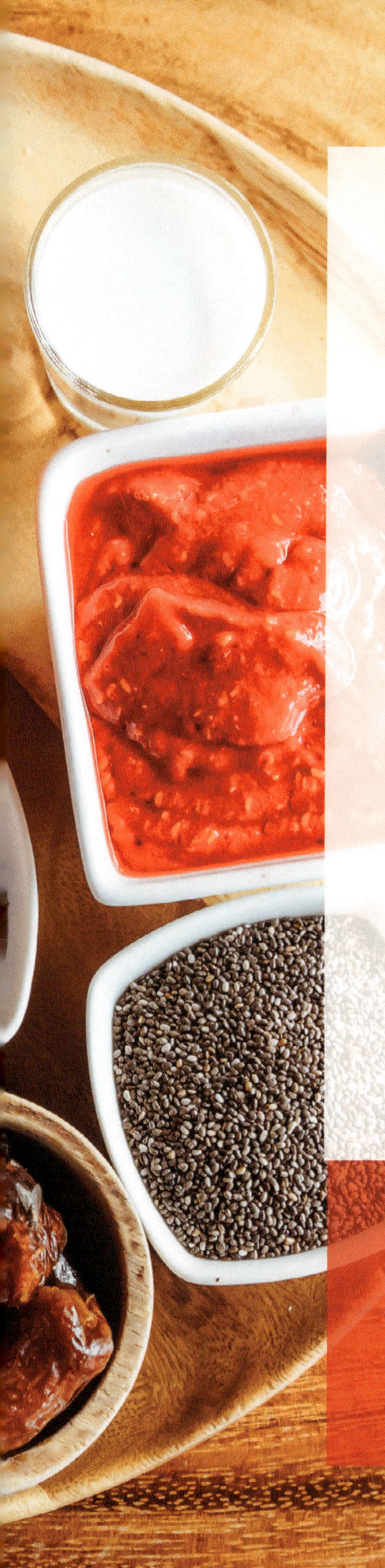

Teasingly tart on the tongue, you'd never guess this fruity potion is packed with fatty acids. Papaya and raspberries form a perfect digestive pair, and the best and brightest of the omegas bond to boost your brain and fill your heart. This one's a rewarding interlude, best enjoyed through small slurps for the most sensory satisfaction.

INGREDIENTS

200 gr Frozen papaya

⅔ cup Hemp milk

½ tbsp Chia seeds

½ tbsp Flaxseed powder

2 Dates

5 tbsp Frozen raspberries

INSTRUCTIONS

Mix all ingredients together in a high-speed blender.

Serving Size: 1
Preparation Time: 5 minutes

Flax seeds provide a major dose of omega-3 fatty acids, making them an essential part of a vegan diet. They also contain far more cancer-fighting lignans than any other plant food. To increase the bioavailability of stored nutrients, grind whole flax seeds just before consumption.

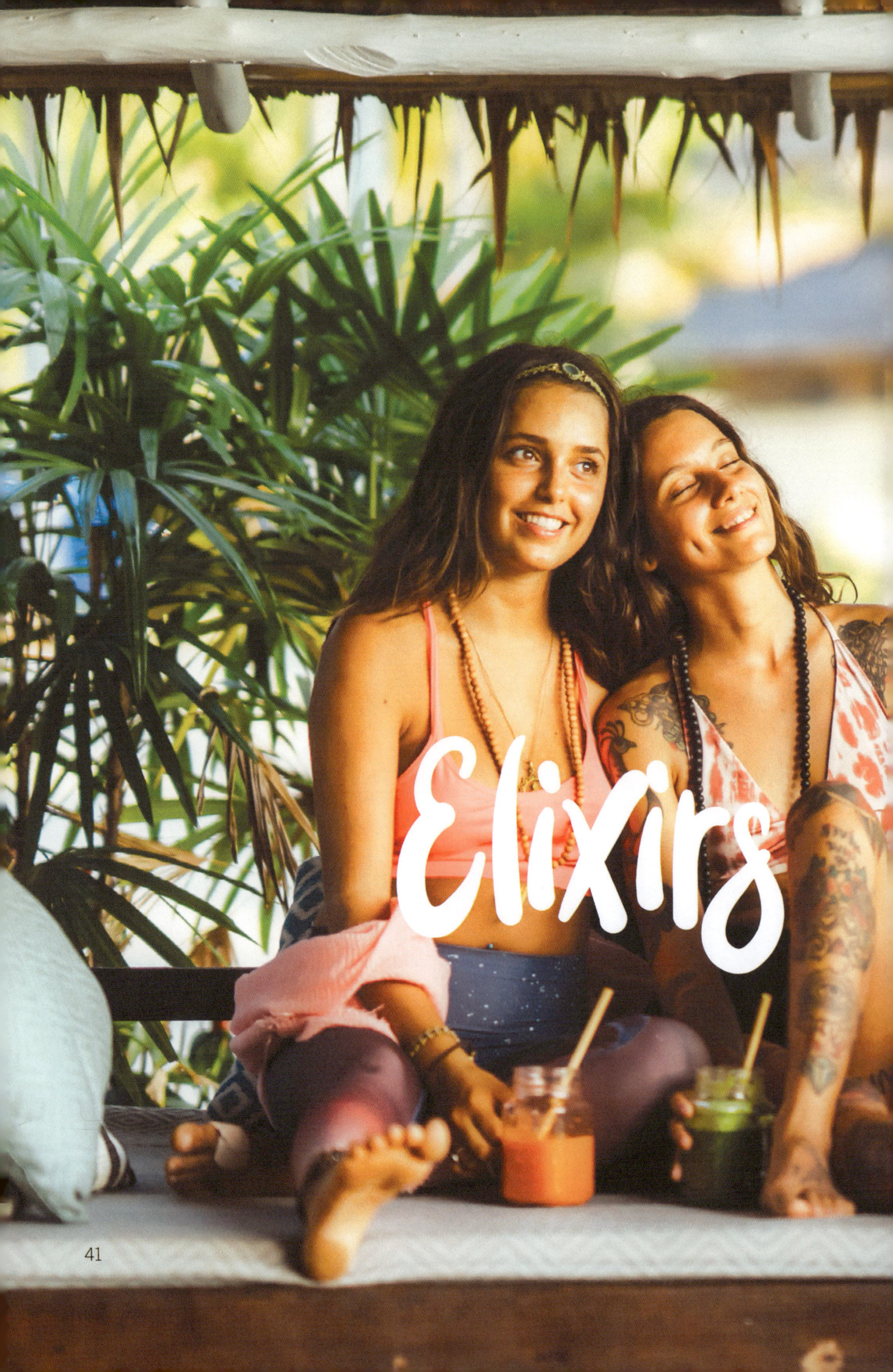

Elixirs

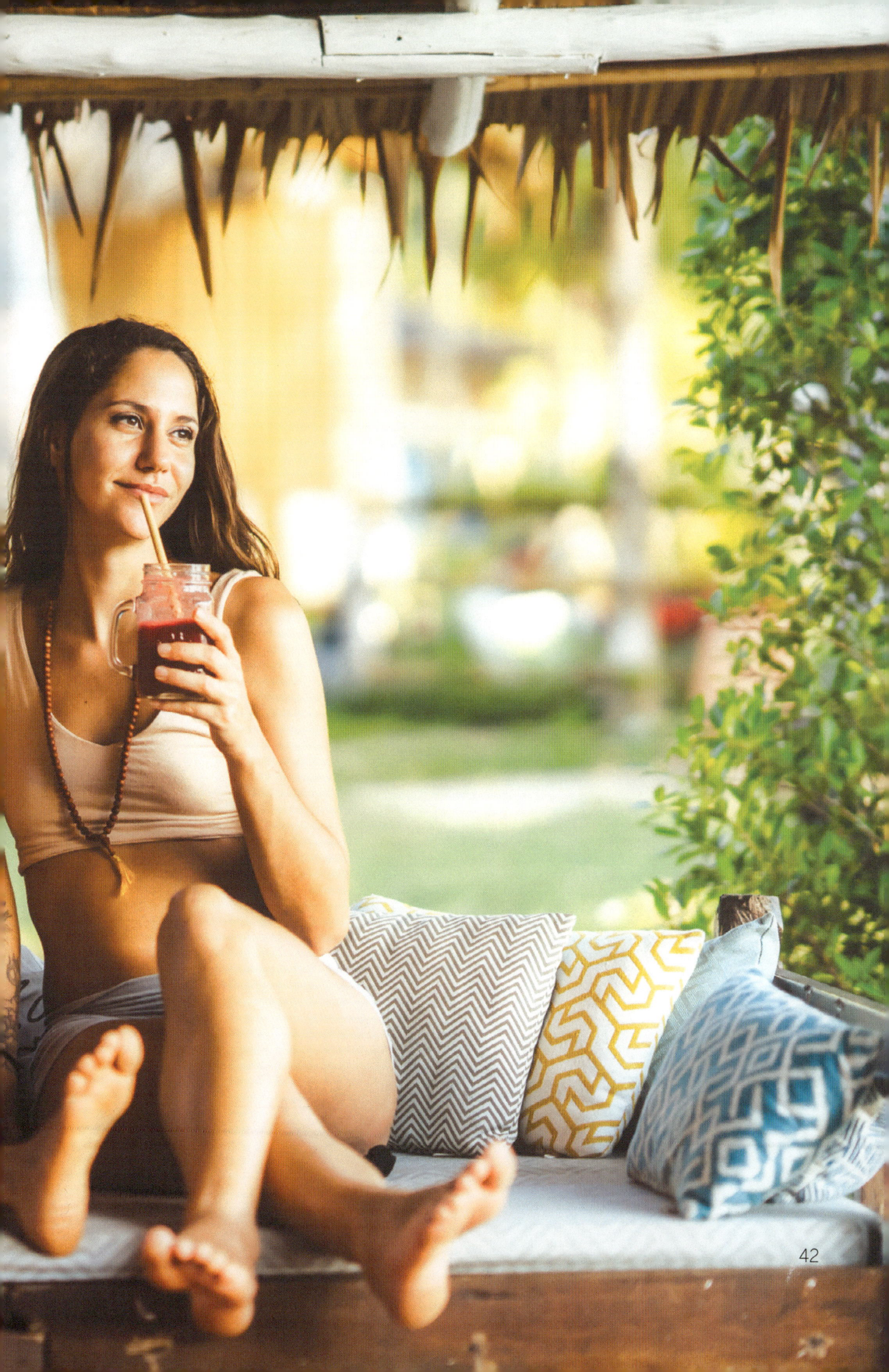

Alkalizer

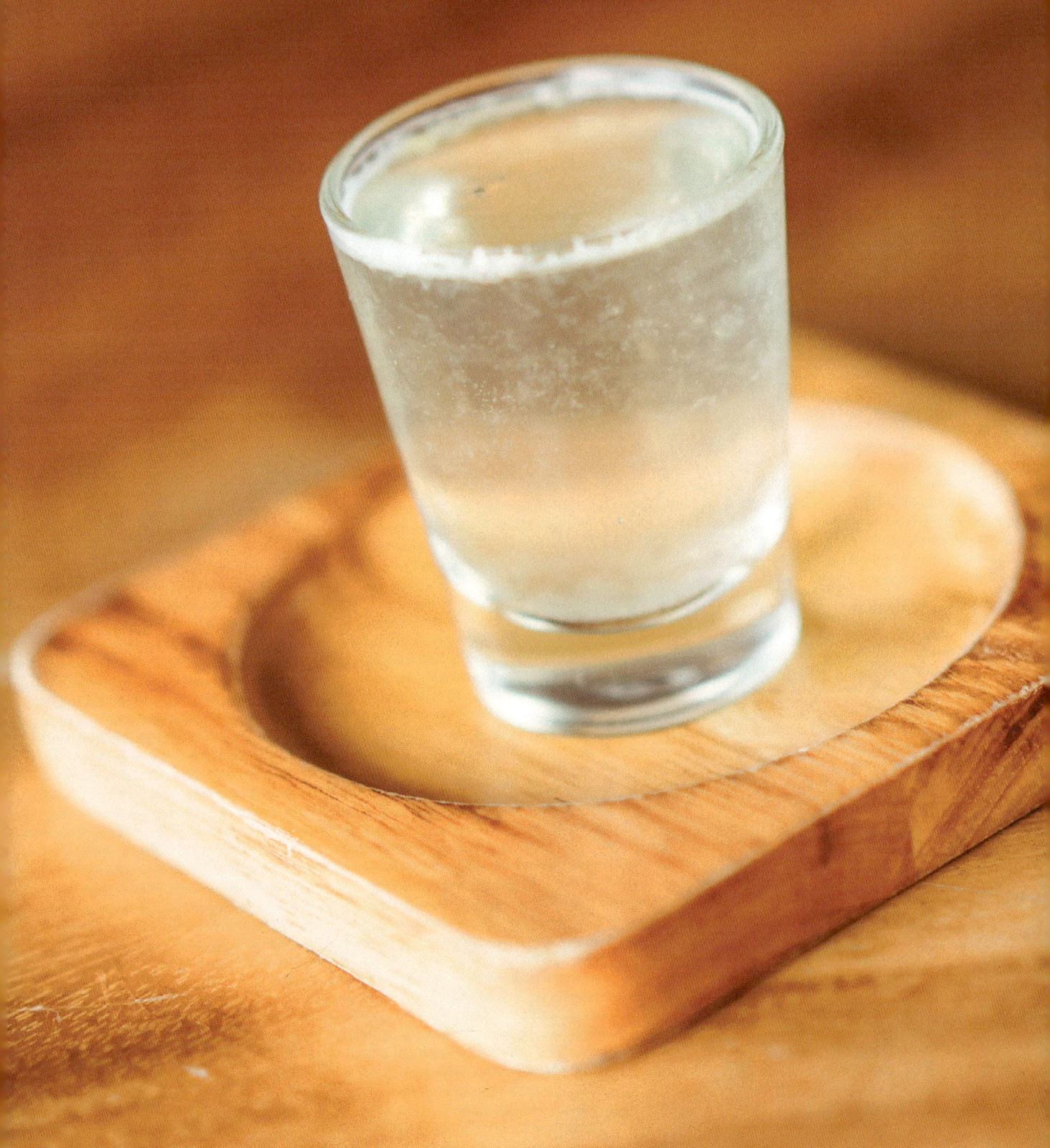

Don't be surprised by the size of this elixir ~ big wonders often come in small shots. This miniature dose of micronutrients gives your gut a warm, salt-of-the-earth reset. Natural electrolytes in Himalayan salt and sodium bicarbonate restore essential minerals and neutralize acids. A squeeze of fresh lime adds a pleasant zing and has an alkalizing effect. Stay hydrated and clear during a cleanse or detox. Enjoy this upgraded shot on an empty stomach for the most powerful benefits.

INGREDIENTS

Juice from ½ a Lime

Pinch of Baking soda

Pinch of Himalayan salt

¼ cup Warm water

INSTRUCTIONS

Squeeze the juice from the lime and stir with a pinch of baking soda and Himalayan salt into warm water.

Serving Size: 1
Preparation Time: 1 minute

Baking soda is alkaline, which makes it a superpower for restoring pH balance and essential electrolytes when dehydration or illness occur. It also helps calm the belly by reducing stomach acid and alleviating indigestion.

Wellness Shot

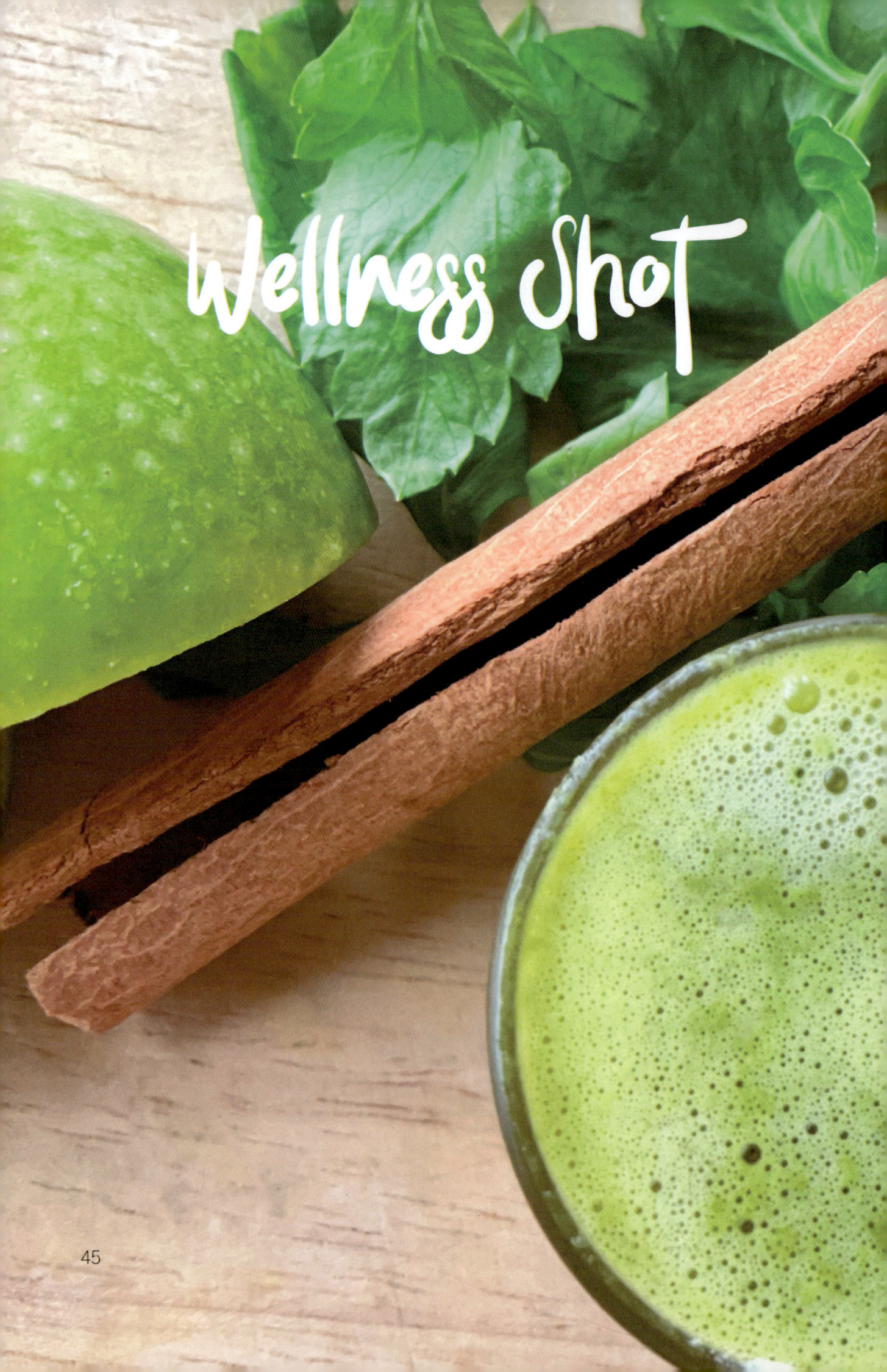

For wellness in body, mind, and soul, feed all three a bit of the earth, the sun, and the spice that gives life its flavour. This grounding, punchy, earthy extract sets your digestive tract right with abundant cleansing micronutrients gifted by celery, lemon, ginger, and a pinch of cayenne. A happy belly is the foundation for zero inflammation and total wellness.

INGREDIENTS

30 gr Celery leaf

10 gr Ginger

1 wedge of Lemon

Pinch of Cayenne pepper

INSTRUCTIONS

Juice the celery leaf and ginger (remove the leaves and use only the celery stalks if you want a less bitter taste). Pour into a shot glass, squeeze in the lemon juice, and add a pinch of cayenne pepper to taste.

Serving Size: 1
Preparation Time: 10 minutes

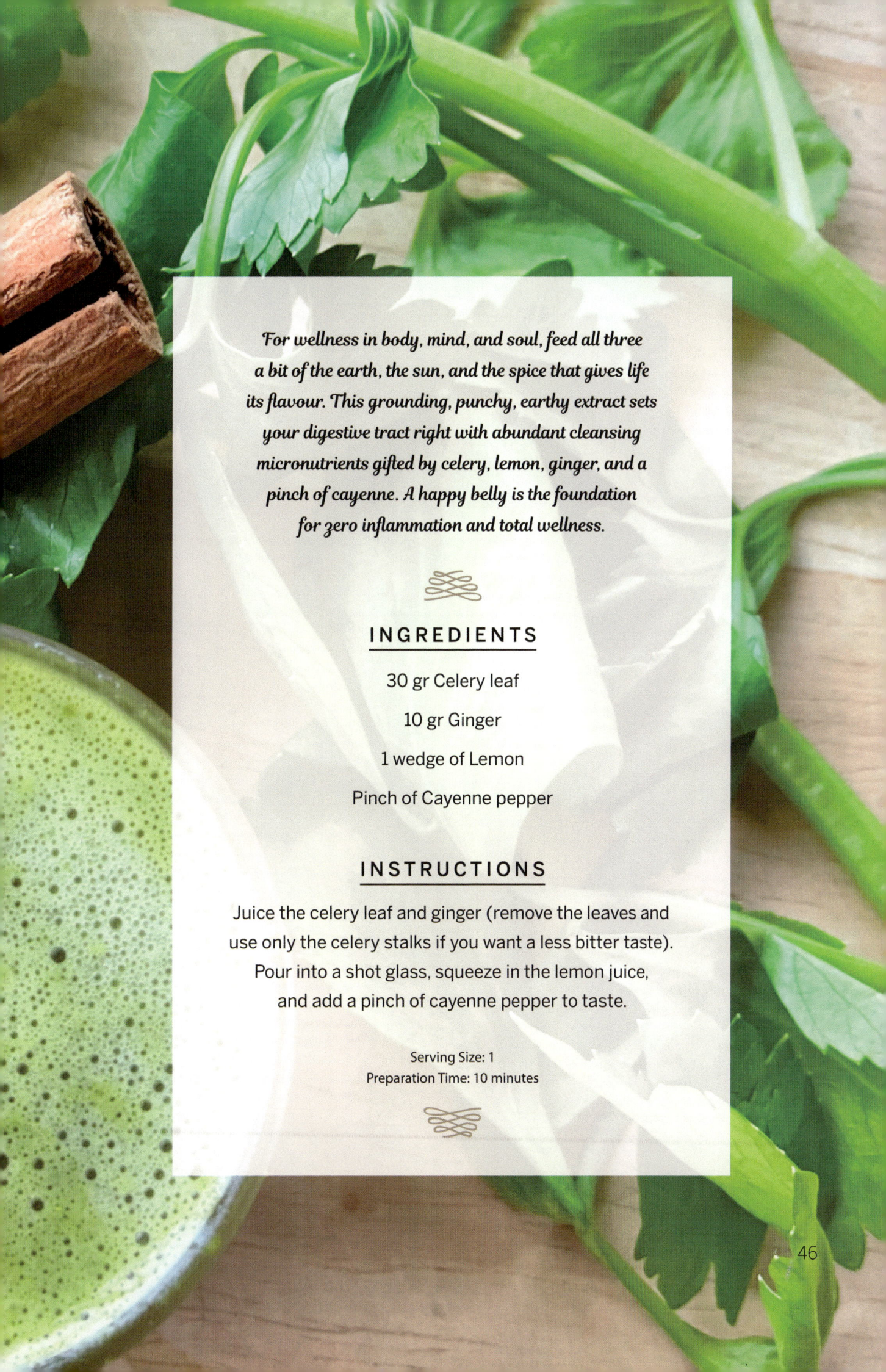

A bit lippy, and wholesomely, sugar-smackingly sweet in a green apple kind of way. Ginger's heat offsets the sweet, and cinnamon offers an aromatic embrace. Loaded with nutrients that combat fungi and candida, this tonic will snap your body's pH back into balance. A daily dose isn't indulgent, it's a health requirement!

INGREDIENTS

50 gr Green apple

10 gr Ginger

Pinch of Cinnamon

INSTRUCTIONS

Juice the apple and the ginger into a small shot glass. Sprinkle some cinnamon on top to taste.

Serving Size: 1
Preparation Time: 10 minutes

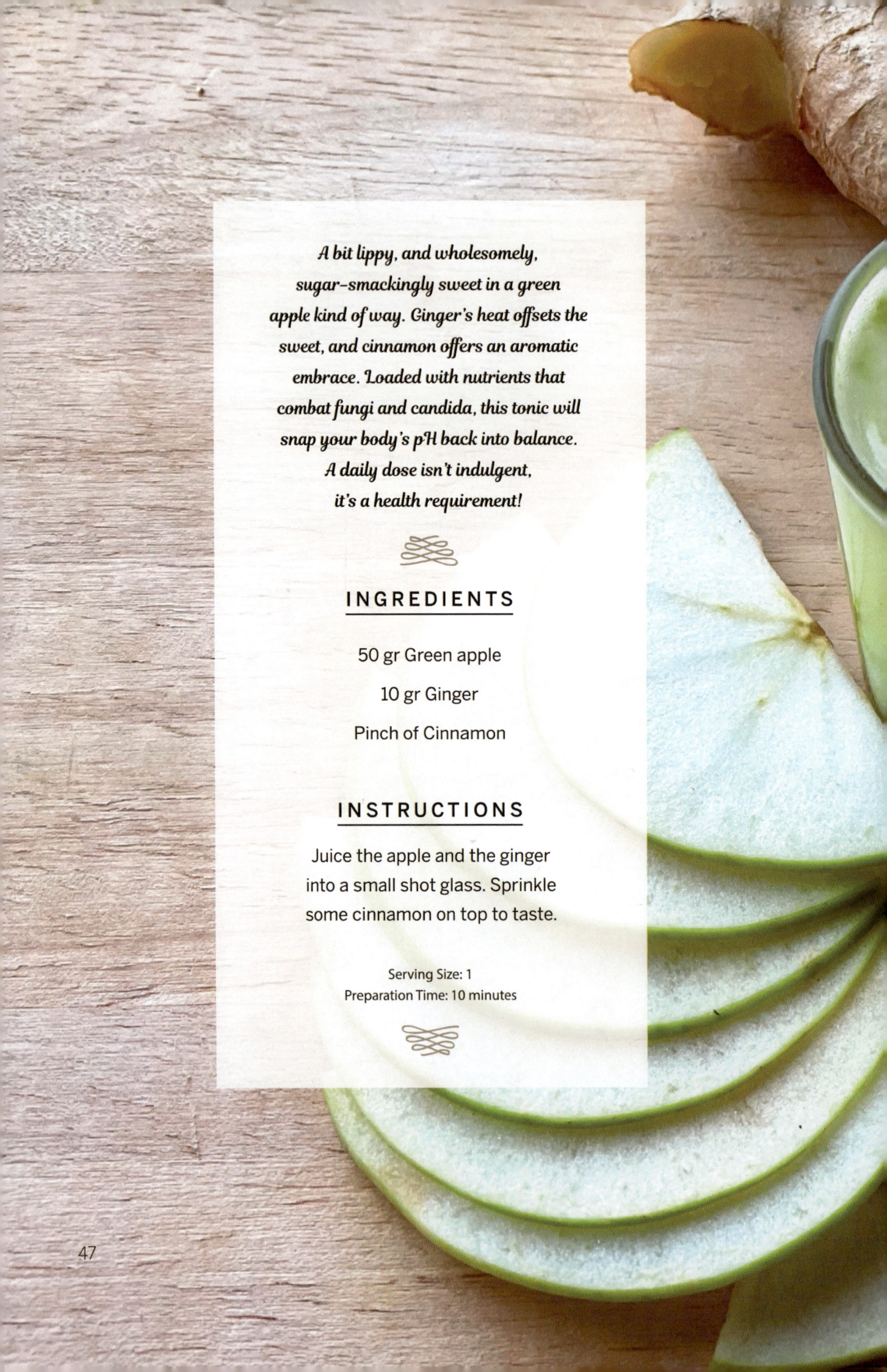

Apple Snap

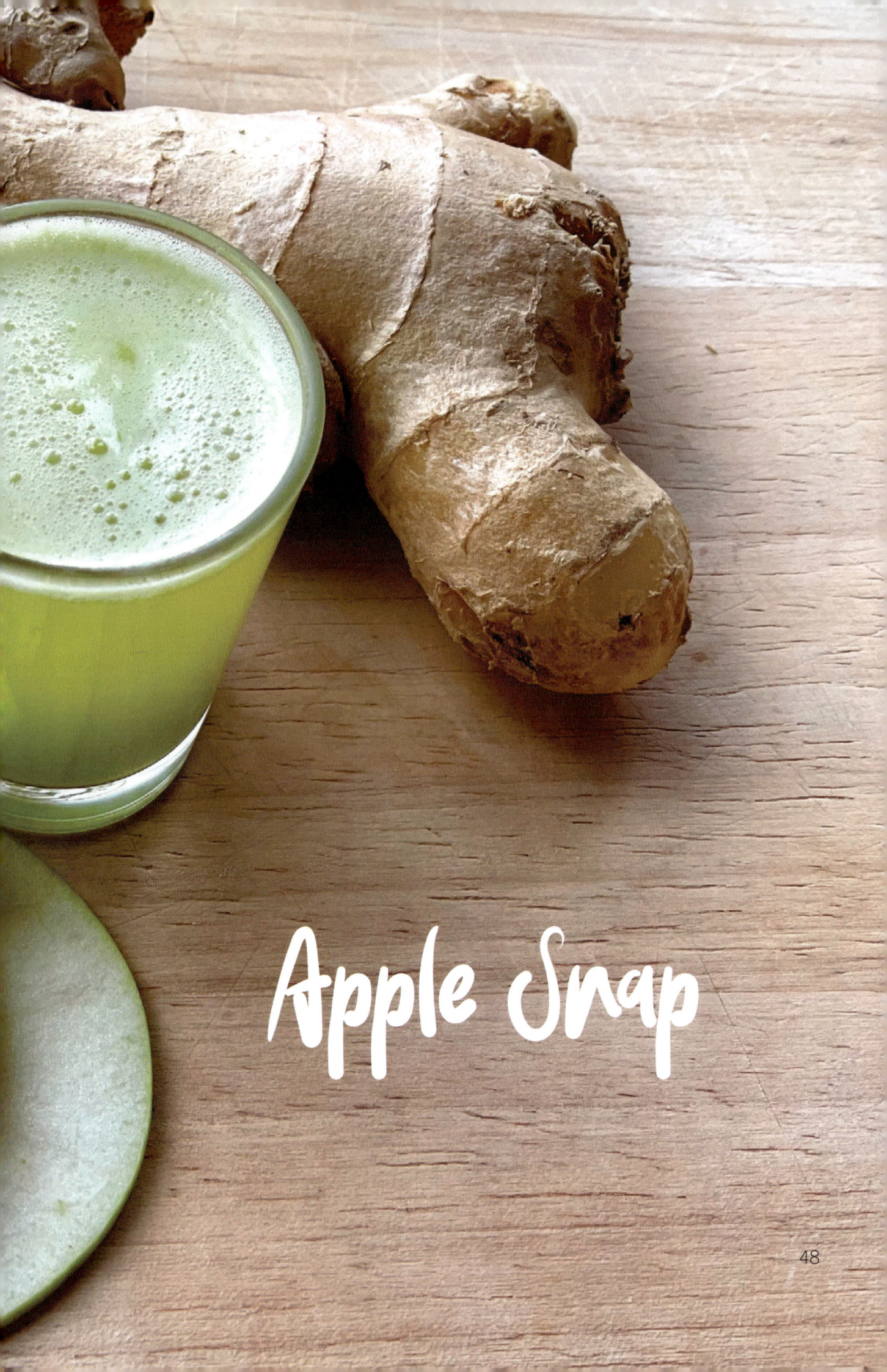

Breakfast

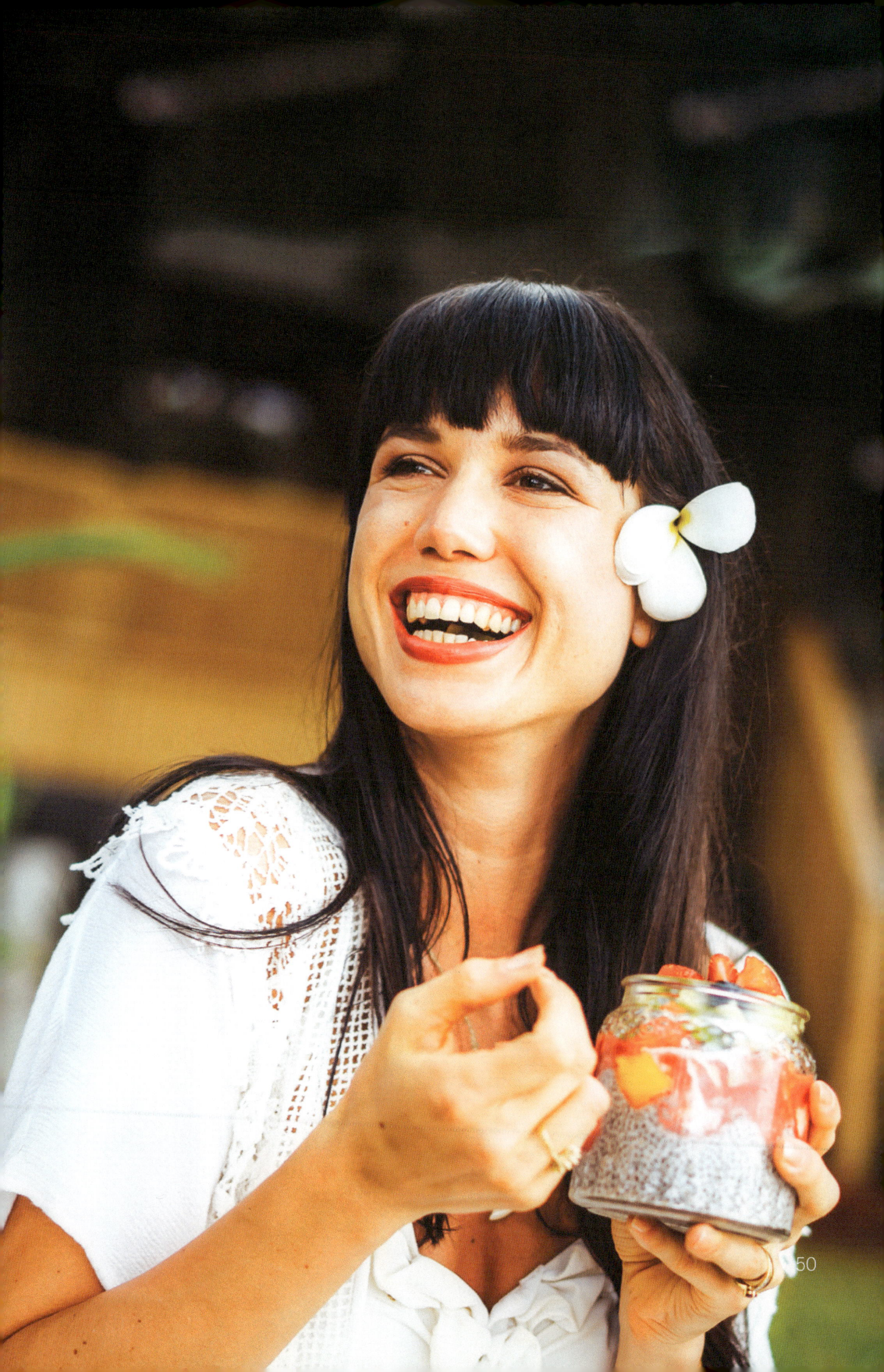

Orion Super Papaya

If papaya wasn't gorgeous enough on its own, its bold acquaintance with dates and creamy tahini enchants even the most hesitant mouth. Sweet, chewy dates nestle into the womb of a halved papaya drenched in thick, rich tahini. A generous sprinkling of freshly ground flax seeds gives a dose of libido-loving fatty acids. Add a squeeze of lime for an island vibe. Enjoy full submission at first bite.

INGREDIENTS

½ Medium-sized papaya

3 Dried dates

½ cup Tahini

1 tbsp Flax seed powder

INSTRUCTIONS

Cut your papaya in half lengthwise, and carefully remove the seeds to create a boat. Chop the dried dates into small cubes. Layer the boat with tahini, dates and top with the flax seed powder. Garnish with freshly squeezed lime juice.

Serving Size: 1
Preparation Time: 5 minutes

Thick, smooth, gently-bitter sesame paste has a variety of uses: as a stand alone dreamy dip, a nutritious thickener for salad dressing, a drizzled topping for fruit salad, and a velvety addition to homemade hummus. Here it balances the sweetness of dates and papaya for a delectable breakfast (or lunch) experience.

Chia Bomb

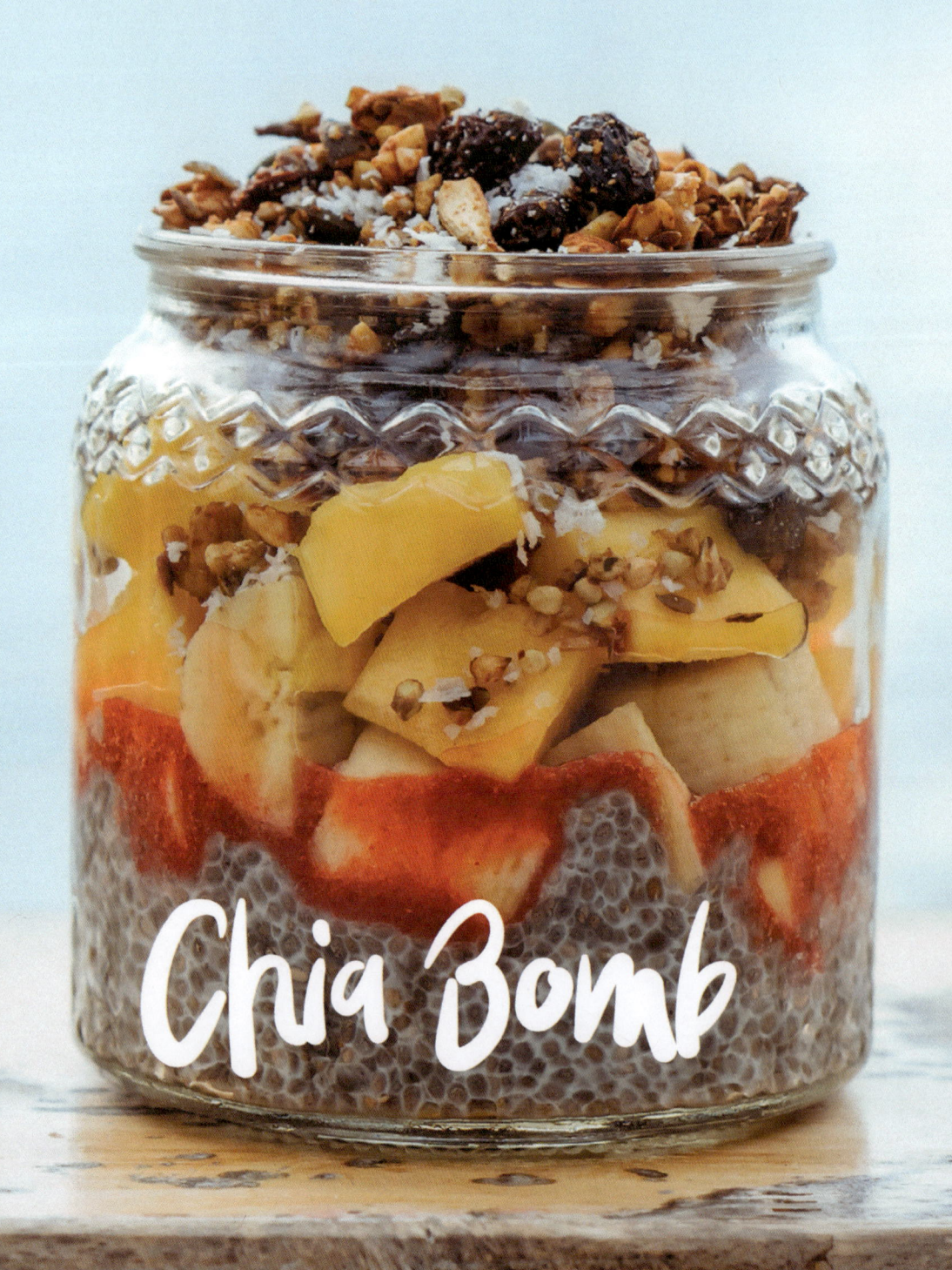

A decadent oasis of sweet berry blend nestled between layers of tropical fruit and slippery chia seeds. Soaking the seeds before mixing with creamy almond milk releases key nutrients and an energy source that opens all the chakras. Garnish with fresh mango, banana, and toasted granola. Dig into this beauty first with your eyes, then with a very big spoon.

INGREDIENTS

CHIA PUDDING

2 tbsp Chia seeds

⅔ cup Almond milk

⅓ tsp Vanilla

STRAWBERRY SYRUP

3 tbsp Blended frozen strawberry

½ tbsp Coconut blossom syrup

Juice from ½ a Lime

GARNISH

1 Mango

2 Bananas

2 tbsp Granola

INSTRUCTIONS

Prepare the chia pudding the night before, or allow the chia seeds to soak in the mixture for 3 hours in the fridge before serving. Stir the chia seeds with almond milk and vanilla, and store in a large jar in the fridge. The next day, prepare the strawberry syrup. Mix the frozen strawberry, coconut blossom syrup and lime juice in a high-speed blender until smooth. Then, garnish the chia pudding base with your favourite fresh fruit. At Orion, we love the combination of mango and bananas. Drizzle with strawberry syrup and crown it with crunchy granola.

Serving Size: 1
Preparation Time: 1 day

Almond milk is one of our favourite fresh milk alternatives and easy to make with the help of a blender. Soaking the almonds is a preparatory step that releases key nutrients, allowing for enhanced absorption. For commercial varieties, check for the organic stamp of approval, and ensure it contains at least 95% almonds and no fillers.

The sweetest of the fruit kingdom unite in harmony in this playful, bright morning breakfast. Smothered in a creamy, tangy coconut yoghurt and topped with a crunchy, nut-based granola, this tango of texture is light, yummy and fresh.

INGREDIENTS

RASPBERRY YOGHURT

3 tbsp Frozen raspberries

3 tbsp Coconut yoghurt

1 Banana

GARNISH

2 Bananas

1 Mango

2 tbsp Granola

INSTRUCTIONS

To prepare the homemade raspberry yoghurt, blend the coconut yoghurt with the frozen raspberries and banana. Pour the yoghurt over a variety of fresh-cut fruits, and garnish with granola or other desired toppings.

Serving Size: 1
Preparation Time: 10 minutes

Raspberries are one of our favourite berries for their sweet and tart flavour, and a colour that will make your heart beam. They're a welcome addition to fruit salad or a blended smoothie, and are chock full of fiber, vitamins, minerals and antioxidants.

Yogi Breakfast

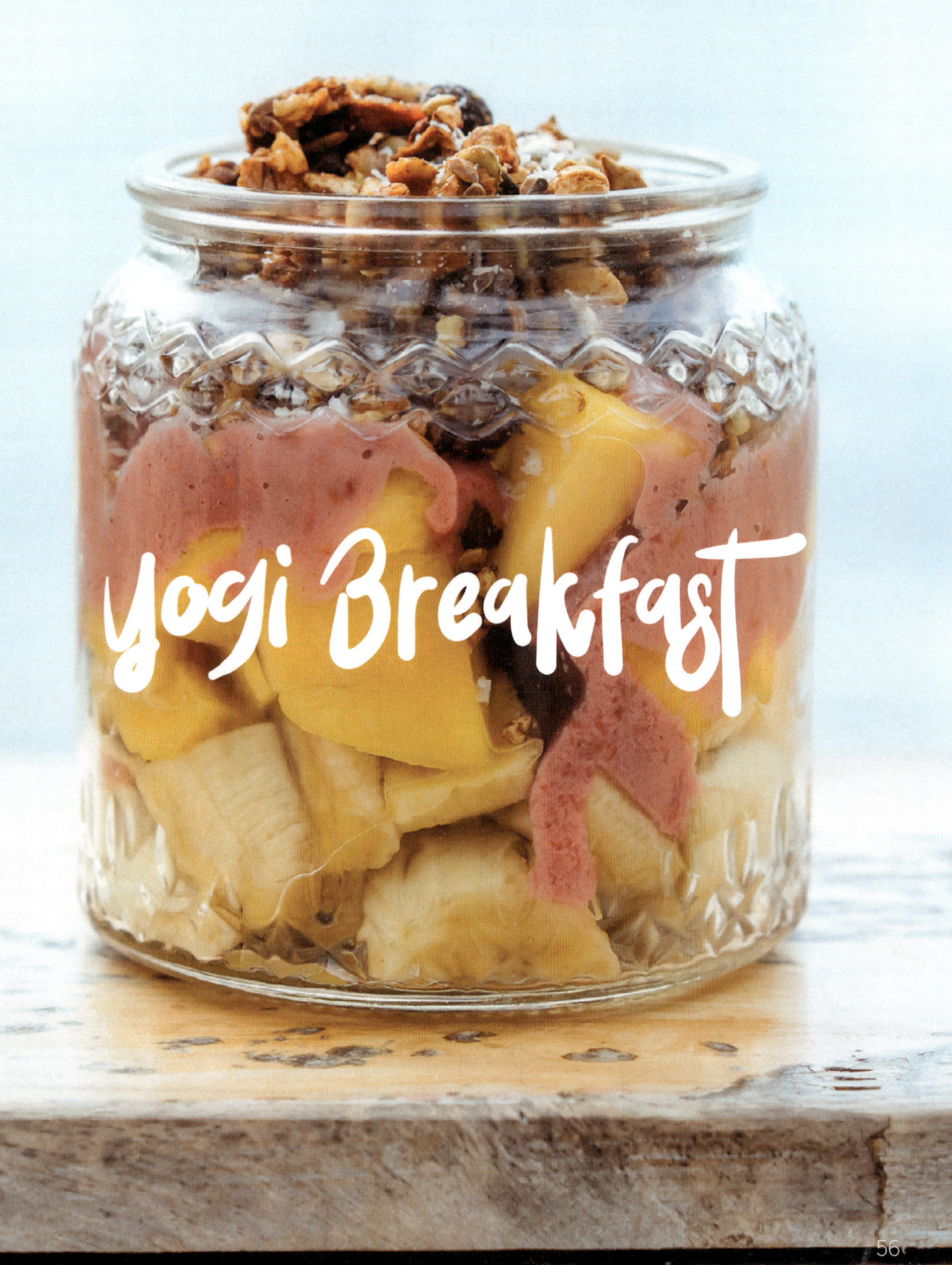

Get your greens on with this hearty, satisfying, and surprisingly easy breakfast bowl that is easily an all-day affair. Don't be misled by the colour – two frozen tropical treats give this green gem an undeniable sweetness and vitality. Sugary date makes a cameo, and coconut puts a bit of meat into it. Made lusciously creamy with fresh almond milk, and topped with the crunchy wholesome goodness of homemade granola, shredded coconut and nuts.

INGREDIENTS

1 Frozen mango	50 gr Coconut meat
200 gr Frozen pineapple	¼ cup Coconut water
5 gr Parsley	¼ cup Almond milk
2 Dates	1 tbsp Spirulina

INSTRUCTIONS

Mix all ingredients together in a high-speed blender. Garnish the smoothie bowl with your preferred toppings, such as granola, dried fruits, shredded coconut and nuts.

Serving Size: 1
Preparation Time: 5 minutes

Another of nature's most blessed offerings comes from the land of palm trees ~ the water inside a coconut is argued to be a more effective hydrator than purified water itself. It's loaded with electrolytes, making it a delicious way to restore pH balance and rehydrate after a long day spent in the sun.

Green Smoothie Bowl

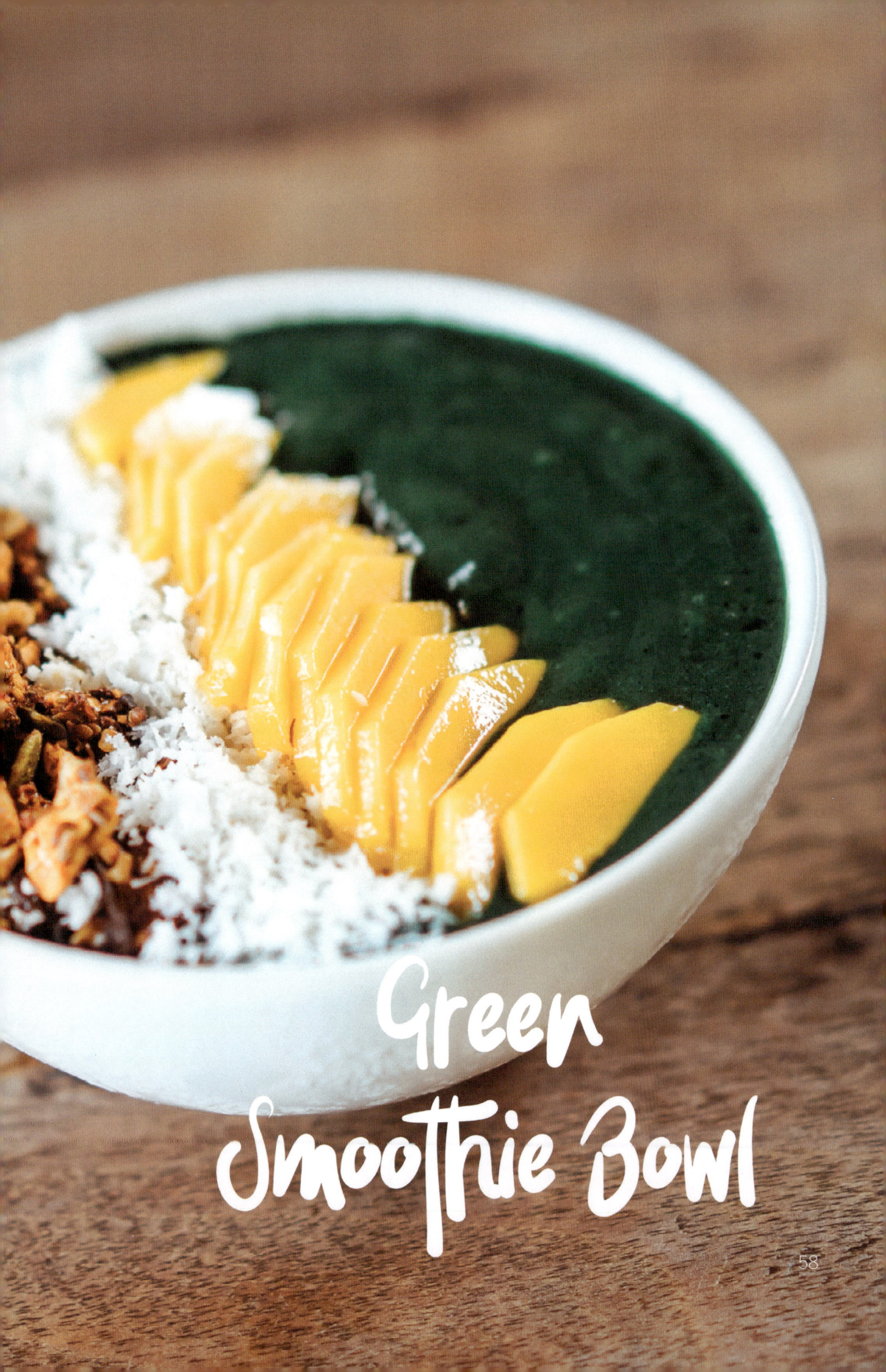

The exact right bite for a hearty appetite. A crepe made from ground chickpeas and nutritional yeast pockets a savoury filling of shiitake mushroom and onion sauté, smothered in tangy, nutty zaatar and soy sauce. Enjoy for breakfast, dinner, or both!

INGREDIENTS

OMELETTE

100 gr Chickpea flour

1 tsp Nutritional yeast

Pinch of Baking soda

Pinch of Himalayan salt

⅔ cup Water

1 tsp Rice oil

FILLING

1 tsp Olive oil

50 gr Shiitake mushrooms, chopped into small slices

100 gr White onion, finely chopped

1 tsp Zaatar

1 tsp Soy sauce

INSTRUCTIONS

Whisk the chickpea flour, nutritional yeast, baking soda, salt, and water together to a smooth batter. Heat the rice oil in a non-stick pan and add the omelette batter. Move the pan so that the batter covers the bottom and forms a circular shape and cook on medium heat for 3-4 mins until the edges set. Flip the omelette and cook until golden on both sides. Keep warm in a low oven while cooking the remaining batter.

For the filling, heat the olive oil in a pan and add the onions, mushrooms, zaatar, and soy sauce. Allow to simmer for two minutes and pour on top of your freshly-made omelette.

Serving Size: 1
Preparation Time: 20 minutes

Also known as gram flour, chickpea flour is high in fiber, folate and other key nutrients, and it imparts a nutty flavour to whatever dish it graces. It's a protein-packed, gluten-free alternative to wheat flour.

Vegan Omelette

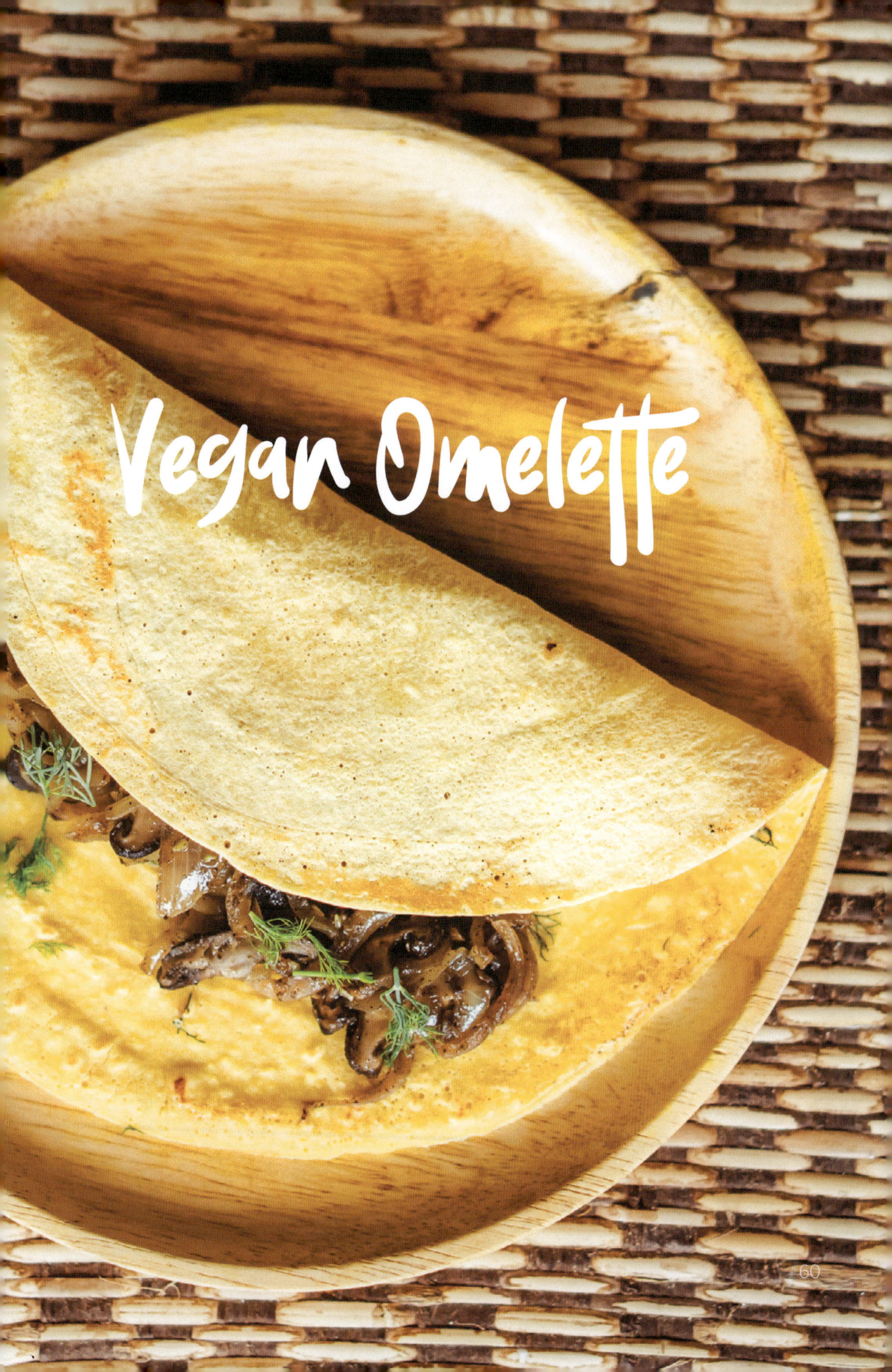

Salads

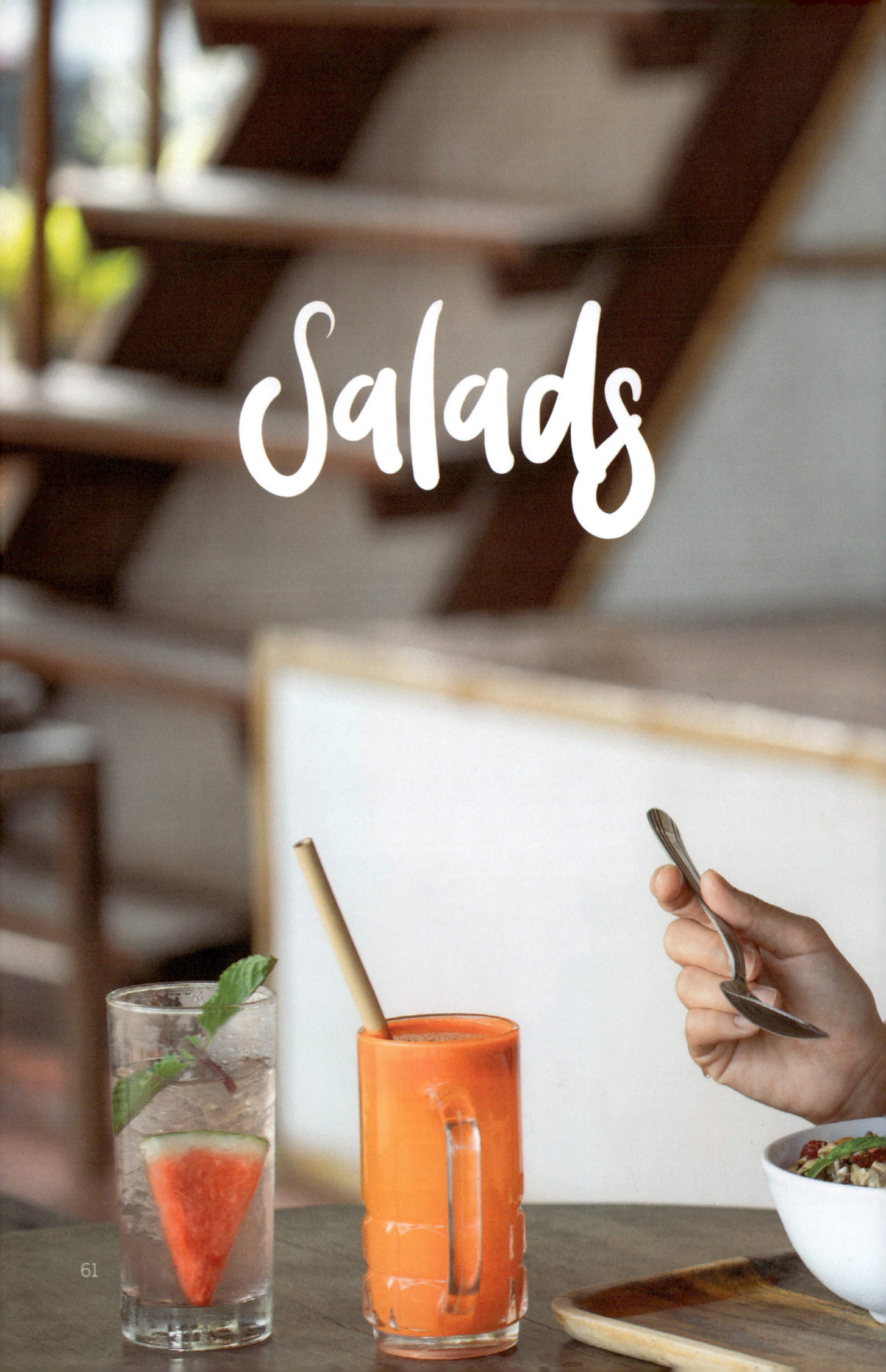

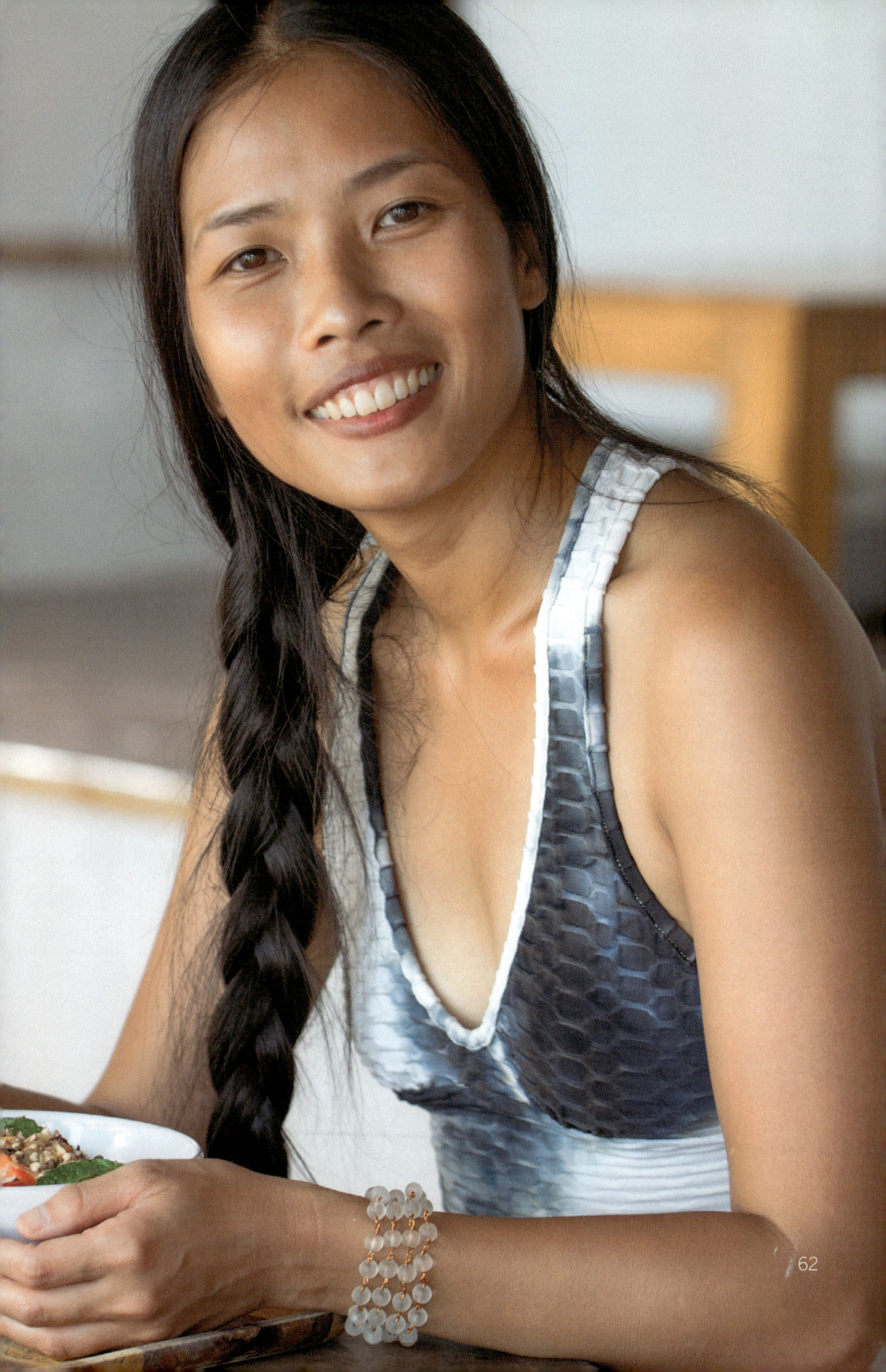

Thai Papaya Salad

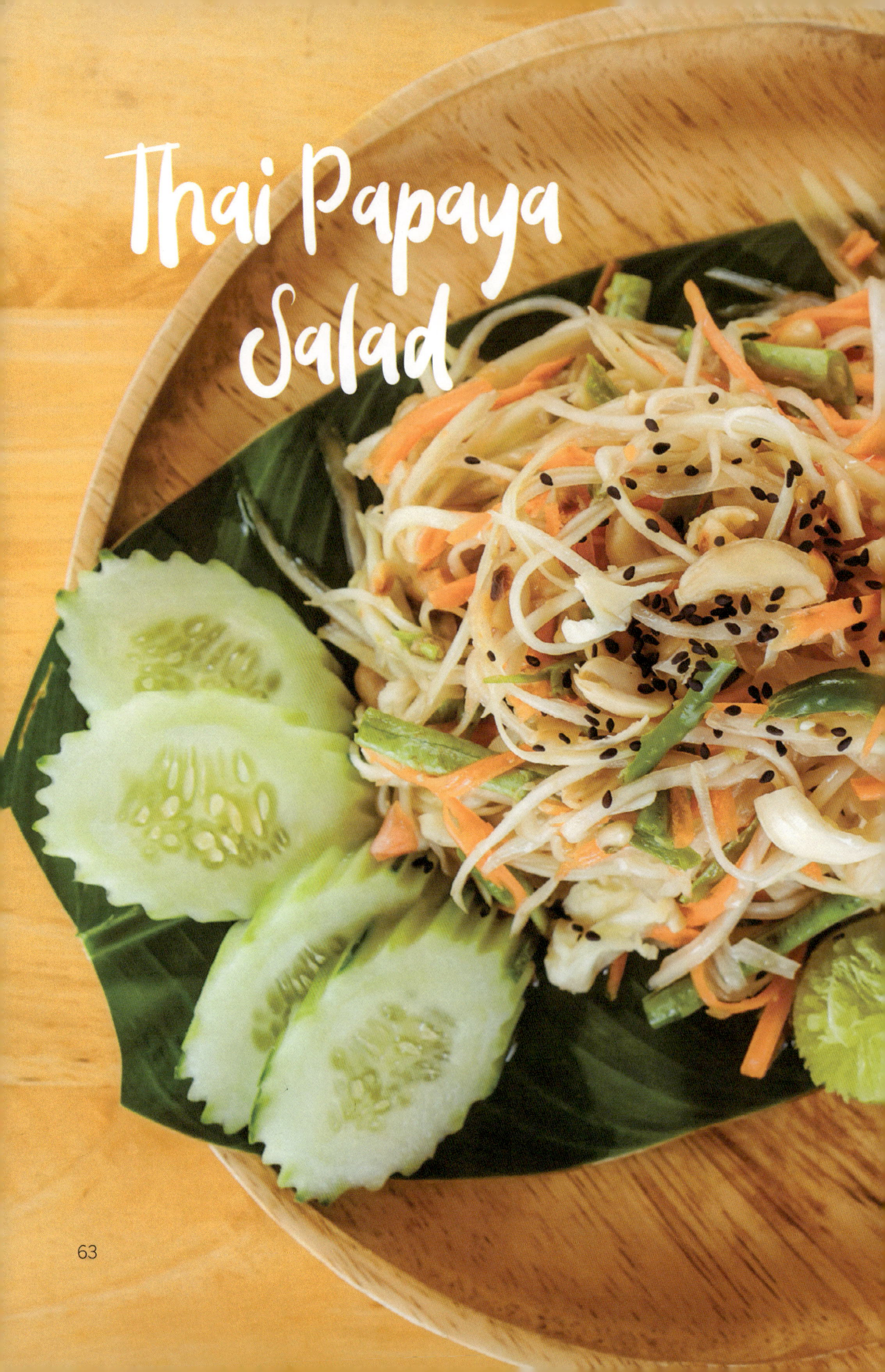

A food stall favourite in Thailand, Som Tam covers the four classic tastes of Thai food in each savoury bite ~ sweet, salty, sour, and spicy. Tomato, garlic, and roasted peanuts mingle amid a gorgeous heap of carrot and papaya slaw. Chillies turn up the heat and Vitamin B-rich long beans raise the vibration. Splendidly crisp and doused in a fresh, delightful tang. Grab a fork and get your munch on.

INGREDIENTS

1 clove Garlic

½ – 2 Red chili peppers
(optional or to taste)

2 tbsp Roasted peanuts (40 gr)

60 gr Long beans (10 cm long)

1 Small tomato (100 gr)

Juice of 1 lime

3 tbsp Soy sauce

⅓ tbsp Coconut sugar paste

50 gr Shredded carrot

200 gr Shredded papaya

What can I substitute for green papaya?
If you cannot find green papaya, don't worry. Substitute with shredded kohlrabi, cabbage, carrots, or bean sprouts. They all deliver the same 'crunch' and carry the dressing well.

INSTRUCTIONS

Traditional preparation of Thai Papaya salad requires a mortar and pestle. In a pinch, use a rolling pin for ingredients such as onions, garlic, or fresh herbs and spices. First, crush the garlic and add the chillies. Then add and crush the peanuts, long beans, and tomato one by one. Next, add the lime juice, soy sauce, and coconut sugar paste. Finally, using two spoons, add the shredded carrot and papaya and mix well.

Serving Size: 1
Preparation Time: 20 minutes

Slow food causes swift attraction. Quinoa is a fiber-rich seed high in protein ~ a surprise, given its weightless airy quality. Bite-sized pieces of dense cruciferous vegetables balance this playful pilaf and add a satisfying, audible munch. Drench with the sensational Orange Olive Oil Dressing several minutes before you eat it.

INGREDIENTS

200 gr Cooked quinoa

25 gr Long beans

25 gr Asparagus

25 gr Carrot

25 gr Purple cabbage

Pinch of Himalayan Salt

Orange Olive Oil Dressing (Page 109)

INSTRUCTIONS

Cook the quinoa and allow it to cool. In the meantime, roughly chop the long beans, asparagus, carrots, and purple cabbage. In a large bowl, combine with the cooked and cooled quinoa and olive oil. Drizzle generously with Orange Olive Oil Dressing and a pinch of salt. Allowing the salad to sit for a while coaxes out the subtle flavours and enhances the taste. Great for the next day's lunch too.

Serving Size: 1
Preparation Time: 20 minutes

Rainbow Quinoa Salad

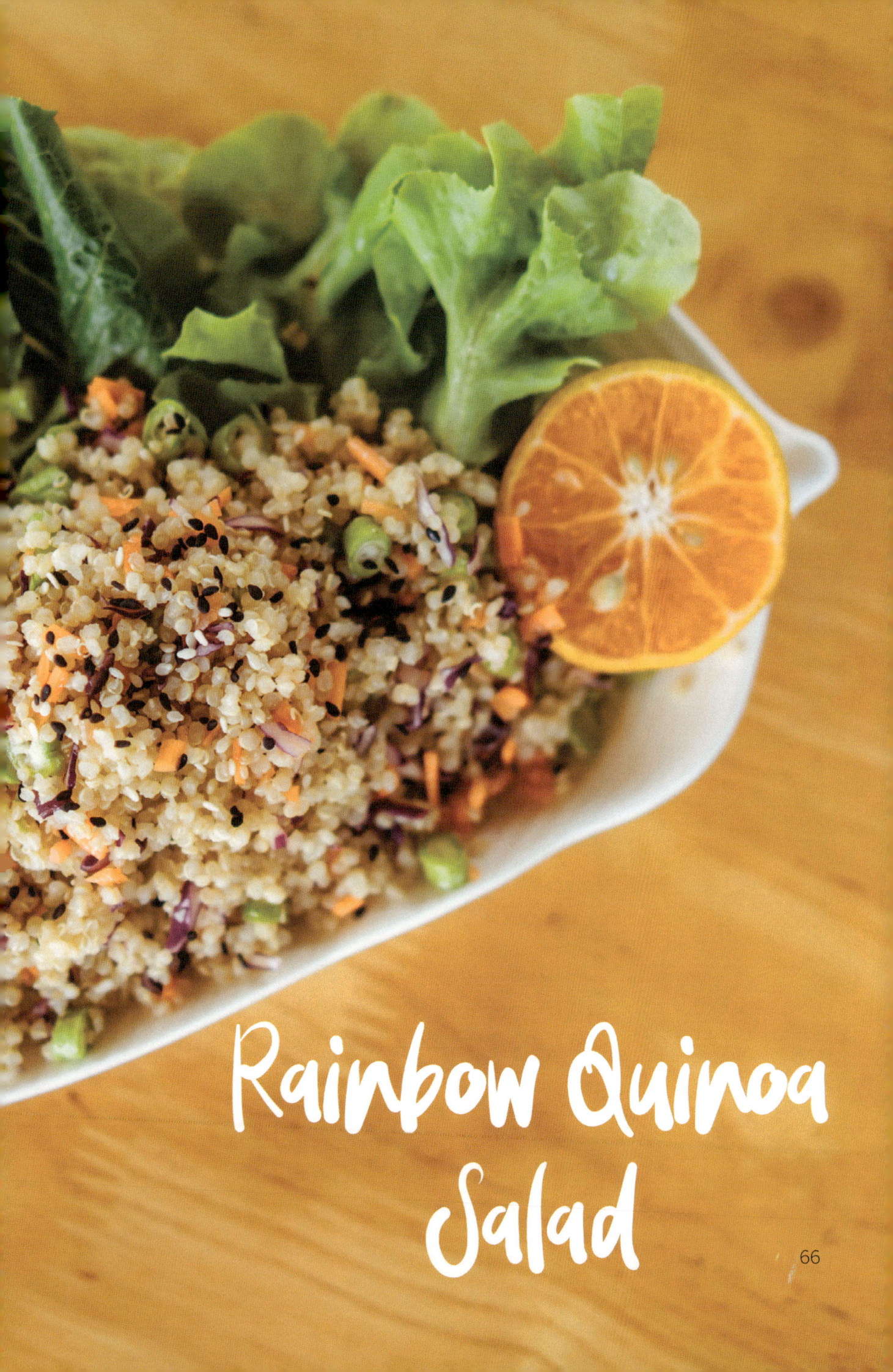

Crisp, creamy, and chewy; all the right textures come together in mouthful after mouthful of this sexy salad. Lashings of Cashew Caesar Dressing seduce crisp romaine leaves into lip-smacking surrender, and tangy sun-dried tomatoes keep you coming back for more. Pair with Raw Seeded Crackers and you'll devote yourself to this one.

INGREDIENTS

1 Medium crispy lettuce

1 Cup Coconut Bacon (Page 134)

1 Cup Roasty Tomatoes (Page 124)

1 Cup Cashew Parmesan (Page 131)

½ Cup Caesar Dressing (Page 133)

1 Handfull of Raw Seeded Crackers (Page 111)

INSTRUCTIONS

Chop the lettuce into rough pieces to keep this dish deliciously crunchy! Pour the dressing over generously, being careful not to soak the salad. Sprinkle with Cashew Parmesan, toss through with Coconut Bacon and Roasty Tomatoes, add a fan of Raw Seeded Crackers to the side.

Serving Size: 5
Preparation Time: 25 minutes

Caesar Salad

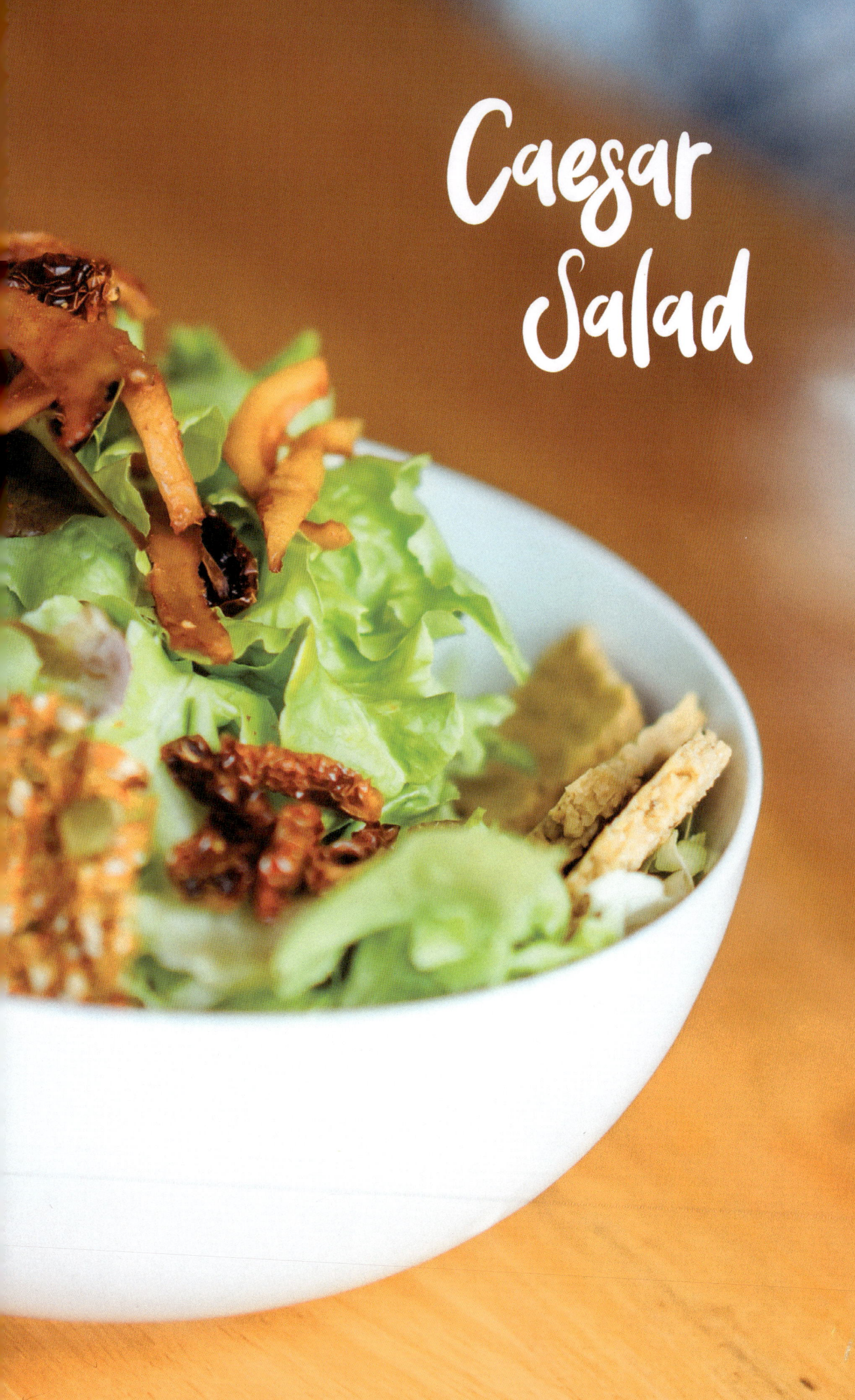

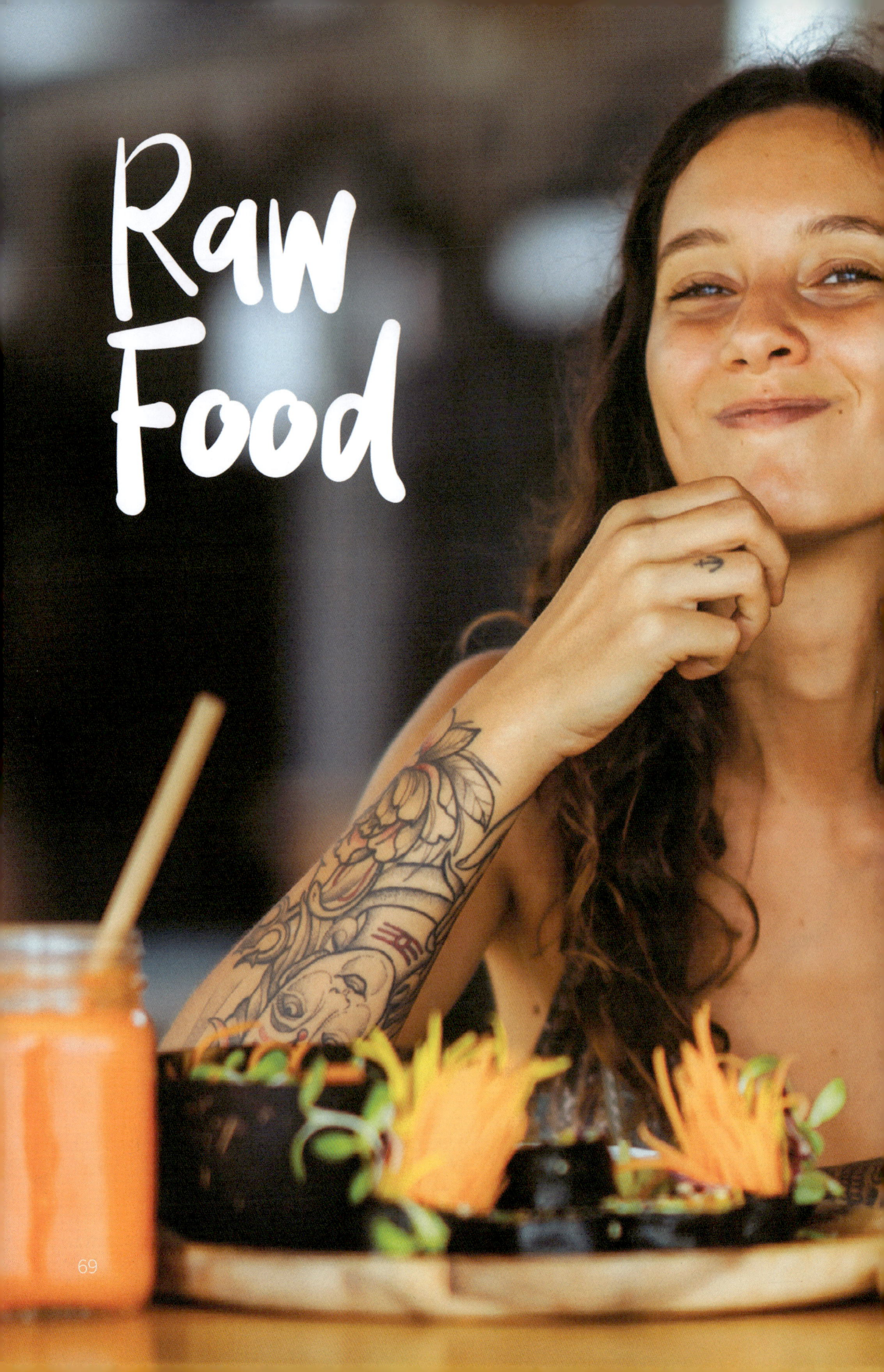

Raw Food

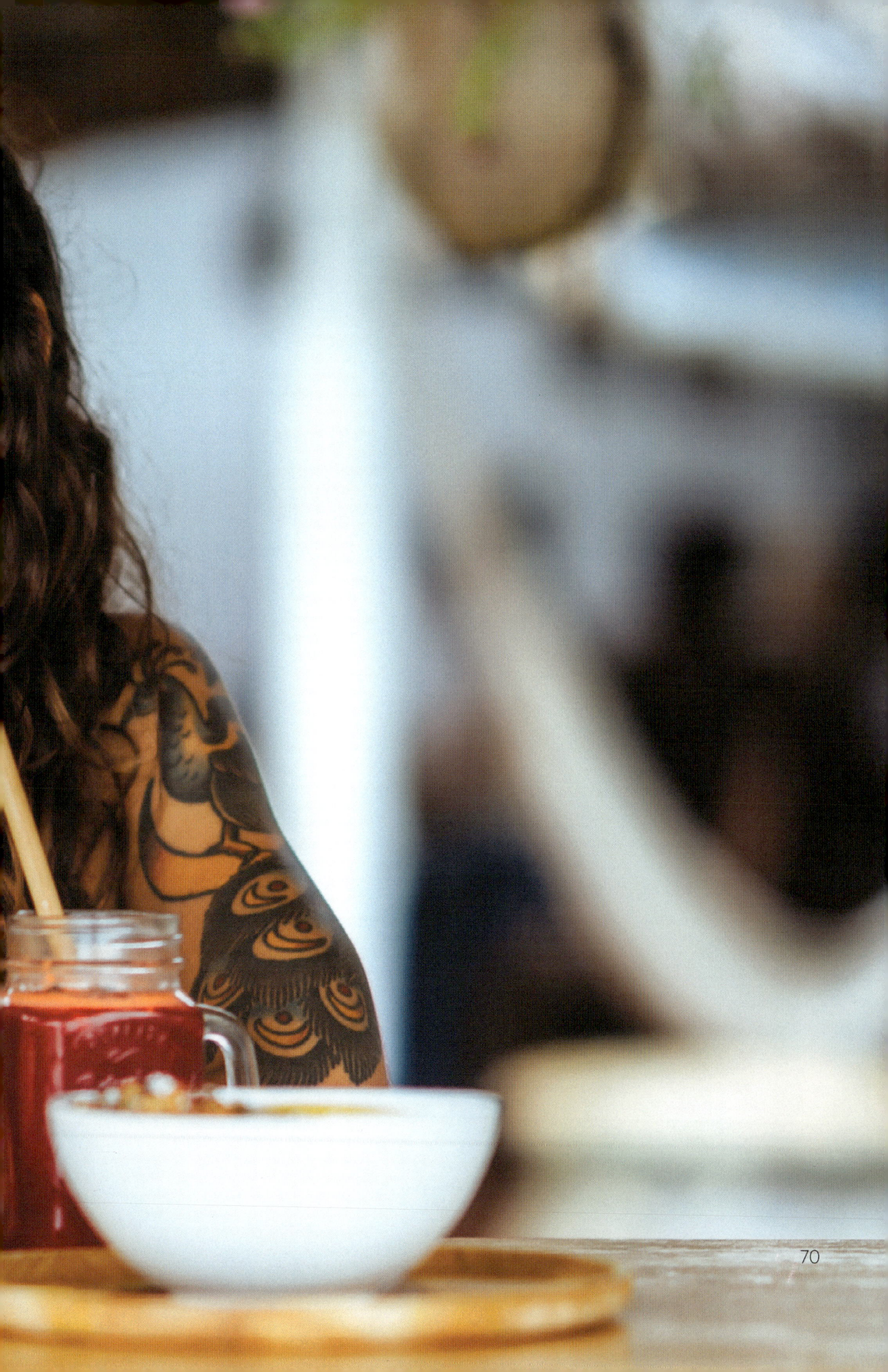

Fragrant and delightfully drippy, this trio of tacos is a handheld masterpiece. Crisp and hearty lettuce leaves cradle a saucy heap of seeds, fresh herbs, and earthy vegetables with rich and creamy Cashew Cheese (see Sauces & Sides) lovingly embracing the whole mash-up. Wrap and roll this finger-licking goodness x 3.

INGREDIENTS

TACO MEAT

100 gr Sunflower seeds

2 tbsp Nutritional yeast

600 gr Carrots

40 gr Spring onion

70 gr Celery leaves

25 gr Fresh ginger

3 Cloves garlic

100 gr White onion

4 tbsp Apple cider vinegar

½ tbsp Himalayan salt

SHELLS & SIDES

8 x 3 Lettuce leaves per serve

100 gr Tomatoes, chopped

20 gr Spring onion, chopped

100 gr Mixed greens

*Cashew Cheese (Page 128)

INSTRUCTIONS

Taco Meat

Blend all ingredients in a food processor. Avoid overmixing, as they will quickly form a paste. Remove the taco meat from the processor and set aside.

Plating

To assemble the tacos, place 2 – 3 tbsp of the taco meat on each lettuce leaf. Top with Cashew Cheese, chopped tomatoes, and chopped spring onions. Serve 3 a portion with a small green salad.

Serving Size : 8
Preparation Time: 45 minutes

Raw Trinity Tacos

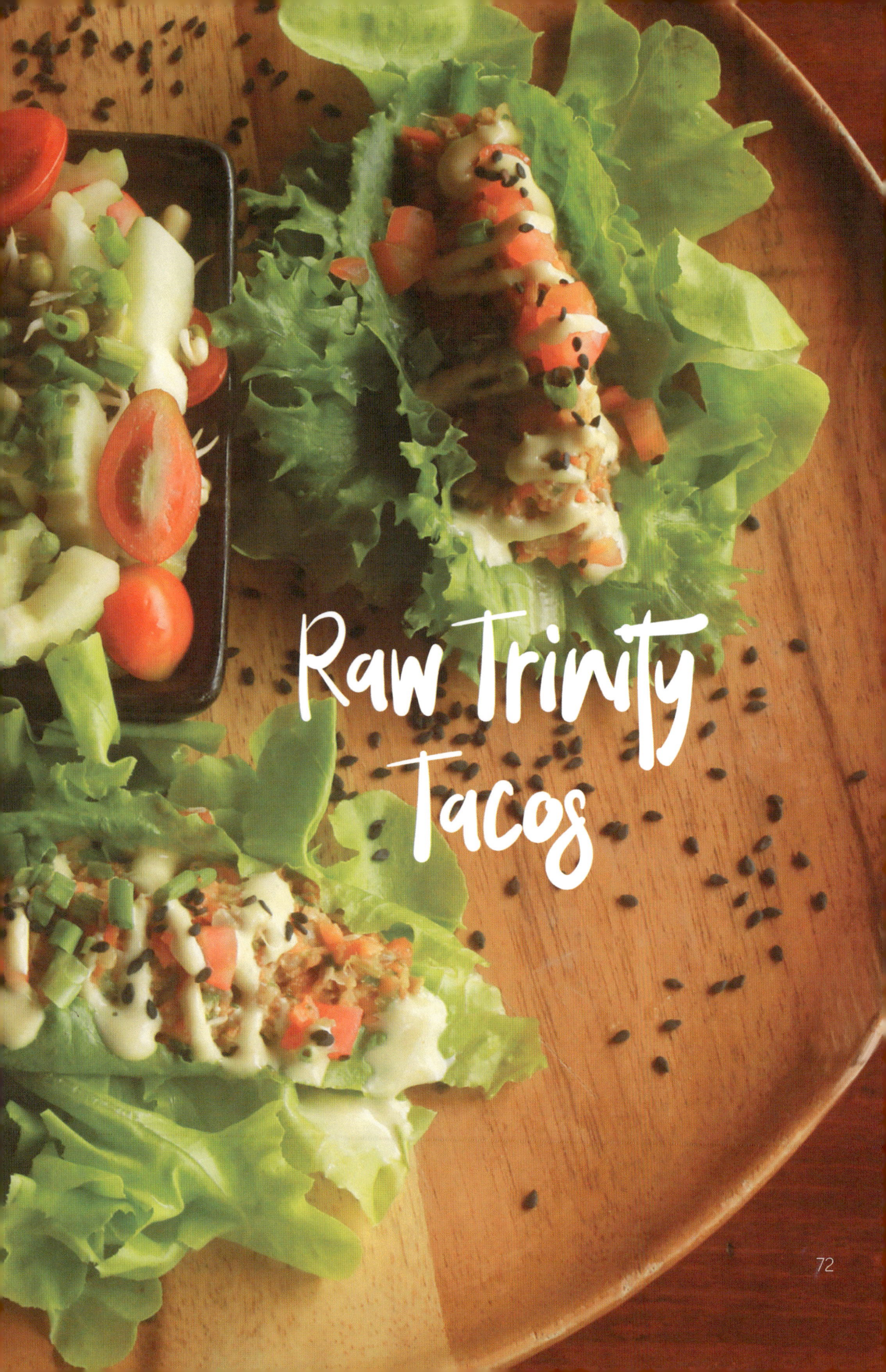

Raw Rainbow Sushi

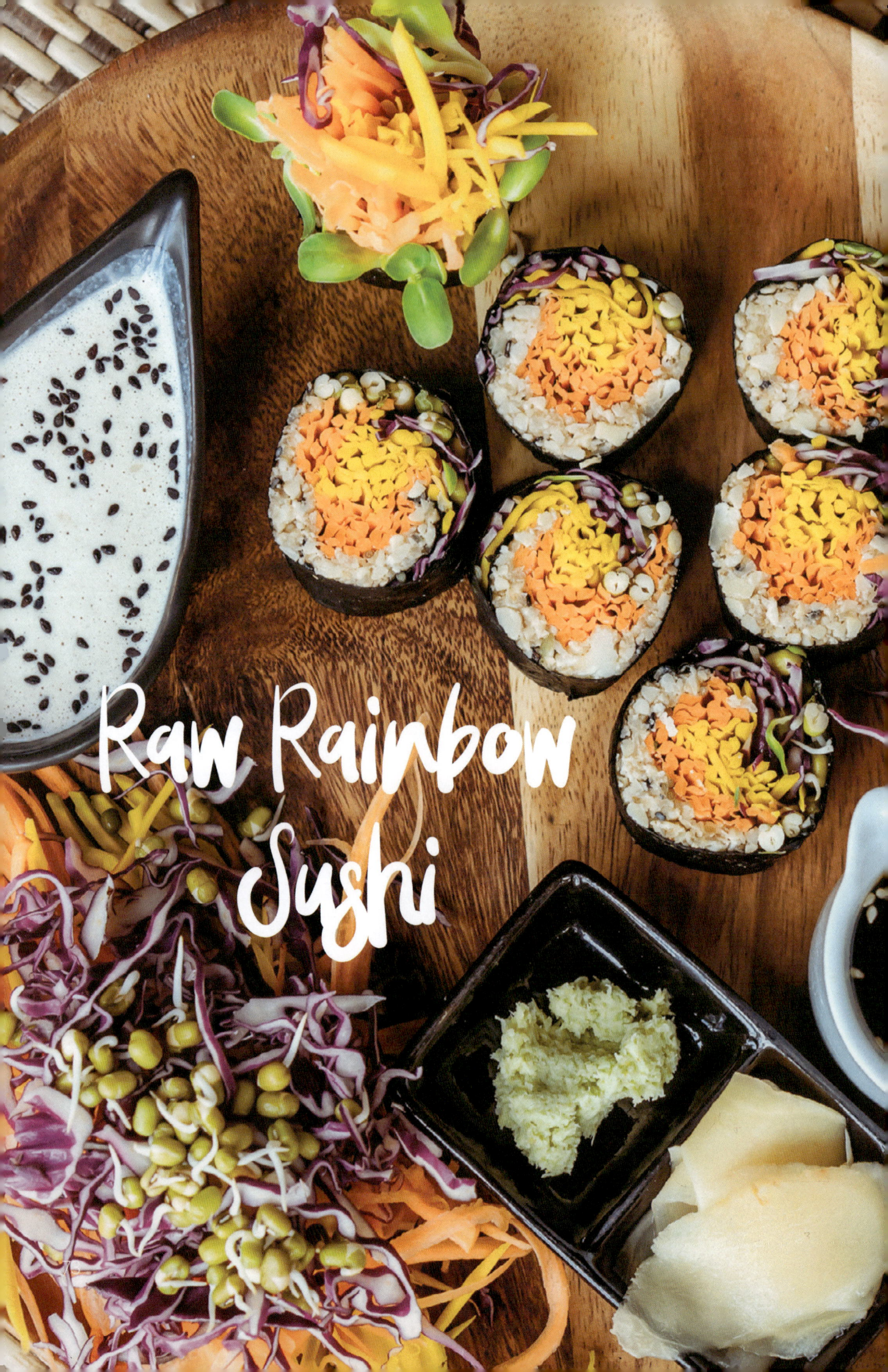

You'll eat this with your eyes. A hand-rolled sensation teeming with crisp, raw vegetables intentionally arranged into a work of edible art. Precise slicing honours each part of the mélange from the slender, snappy carrot sticks to strips of purple cabbage and raw pumpkin straws. A slight taming of hearty sprouts is required. Decimated cauliflower and cashew nuts unite on paper-thin nori and form the bed on which it all rolls up into a rainbow of colour and crunch. Slice into bite-sized pieces to expose the magic of intentional creation. Enjoy with drippings of Soy Sesame Dressing, fresh wasabi, and pickled ginger.

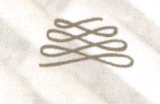

INGREDIENTS

Sushi Rice

50 gr Cashew nuts

400 gr Raw cauliflower

2 tbsp Olive oil

30 gr Black sesame seeds

Filling

2 Small carrots, thinly sliced

1 Medium purple cabbage, thinly sliced

100 gr Pumpkin, thinly sliced

100 gr Sunflower sprouts

6 tbsp Mung bean sprouts

Plating

Nori sheets

10 gr Pickeled ginger

Wasabi

Green salad

Soy Sesame Dressing

(Page 118)

INSTRUCTIONS

Blend the cashew nuts in a food processor, and set aside. Blend the raw cauliflower in the food processor. Avoid overmixing so the texture remains crunchy and has the size and texture of rice. Using two spoons, carefully mix the cauliflower and the cashew nut together, then add the olive oil, Himalayan salt, and sesame seeds. Place the nori sheet on a clean surface, gently and evenly spread the sushi rice to cover the nori. Arrange the vegetable straws and sprouts on the edge of the sushi rice. Then gently roll the nori sheet tucking in the edge until it's fully rolled up. Seal the roll with a sprinkle of warm water at the ends. Gently cut the roll into small round pieces and serve with a green salad, Soy Sesame Dressing, pickled ginger and wasabi.

Serving Size: 8
Preparation Time: 45 minutes

Tender, hollowed out zucchini boats cradle savoury Cashew Basil Pesto, alight with fragrance and zest. A medley of onions, shiitake mushrooms, and plump cherry tomatoes adds a hearty bite that will make you want to cosy up inside a blanket fort with your favourite person. Drizzle with olive oil and a sprinkle of coarse rock salt ~ the zucchini boats that is, not your friend!

INGREDIENTS

1 Medium zucchini

Pinch of Himalayan salt

½ Onion, julienned

5 Fresh shiitake mushrooms, finely sliced

5 Fresh cherry tomatoes, sliced

2 tbsp Olive oil

A handful of chopped Parsley

Cashew Basil Pesto (Page 132)

INSTRUCTIONS

Preheat the oven to 205°C, and line a cooking tray with parchment paper. Cut the zucchini lengthwise into halves, then trim off the stem ends. Using a spoon, carefully scoop out the flesh to create two boats. Sprinkle some salt on the zucchini halves and place them on the baking tray. Spread some Cashew Basil Pesto on each half and top with sliced white onions, mushrooms, and cherry tomatoes. Drizzle with olive oil. Bake for 15 – 20 minutes until the zucchini is tender. Sprinkle with chopped parsley and serve.

Serving Size: 1
Preparation Time: 30 minutes

Zucchini Friendships

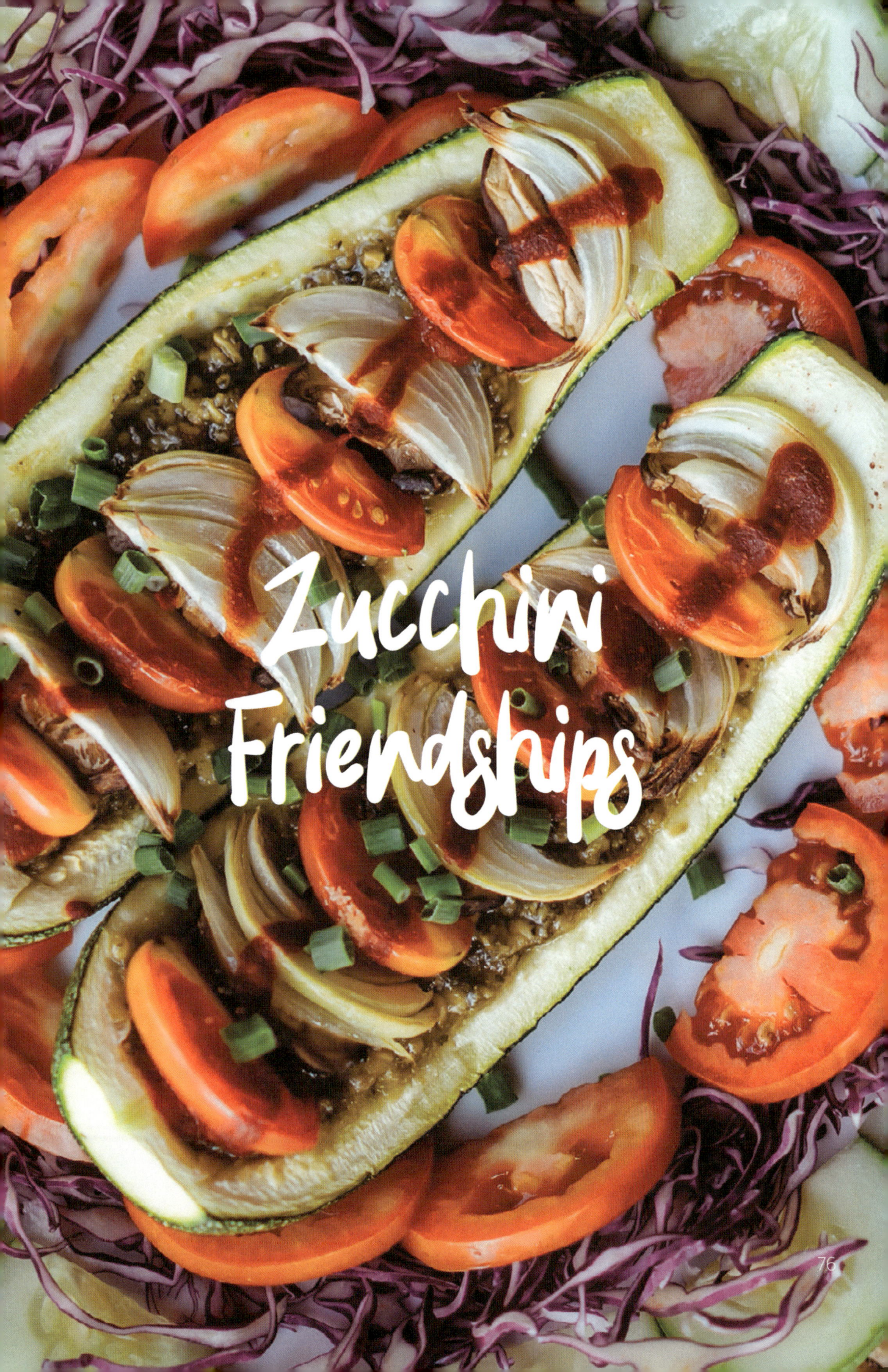

A gratifying heap of raw, crunchy cauli is one of the best ways to cleanse the belly and the spirit, especially when Kale Pesto shows up. This herbed, peppered, and cherry tomato-topped pilaf reminds us of the joy of eating, of tasting each textured bite like it's the first. Make this a main or a side, and rediscover the edible gifts of simple garden vegetables.

INGREDIENTS

350 gr Raw cauliflower

50 gr Red bell pepper, chopped into bite-size cubes

70 gr Cherry tomatoes, cut into halves

1 tbsp Spring onion, finely chopped

1 tbsp Coriander leaf, finely chopped

1 tbsp Parsley, finely chopped

1 tbsp Olive oil

½ tsp Himalayan salt

Kale Pesto (Page 123)

INSTRUCTIONS

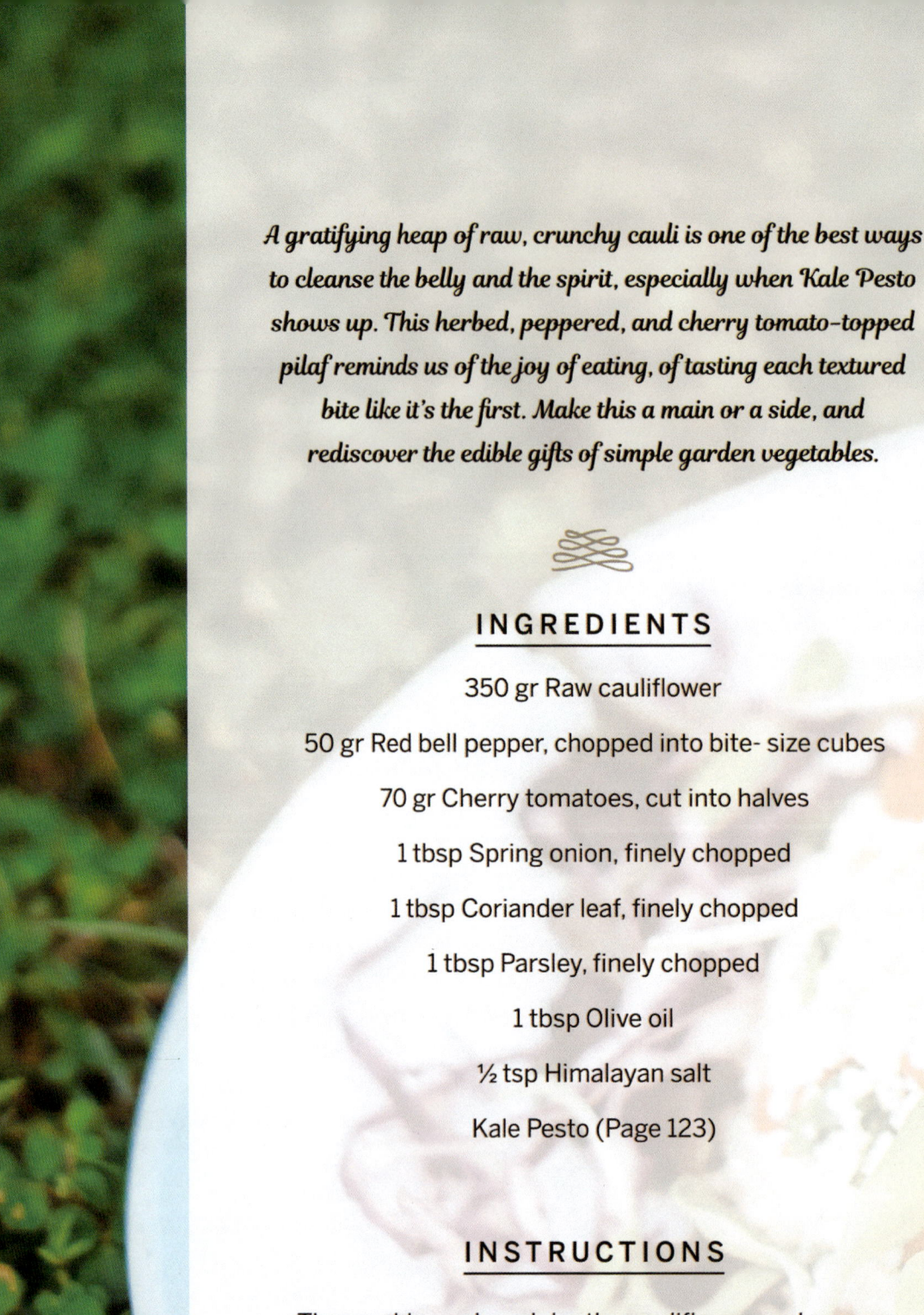

Thoroughly wash and dry the cauliflower, and remove the stem and leaves. Cut the cauliflower into large chunks and grate into rice. Transfer into a big bowl and mix with the bell pepper, cherry tomatoes, spring onions, coriander leaves, parsley, olive oil, and salt. Top or serve with Kale Pesto.

Serving Size: 1
Preparation Time: 30 minutes

Raw Cauliflower Rice

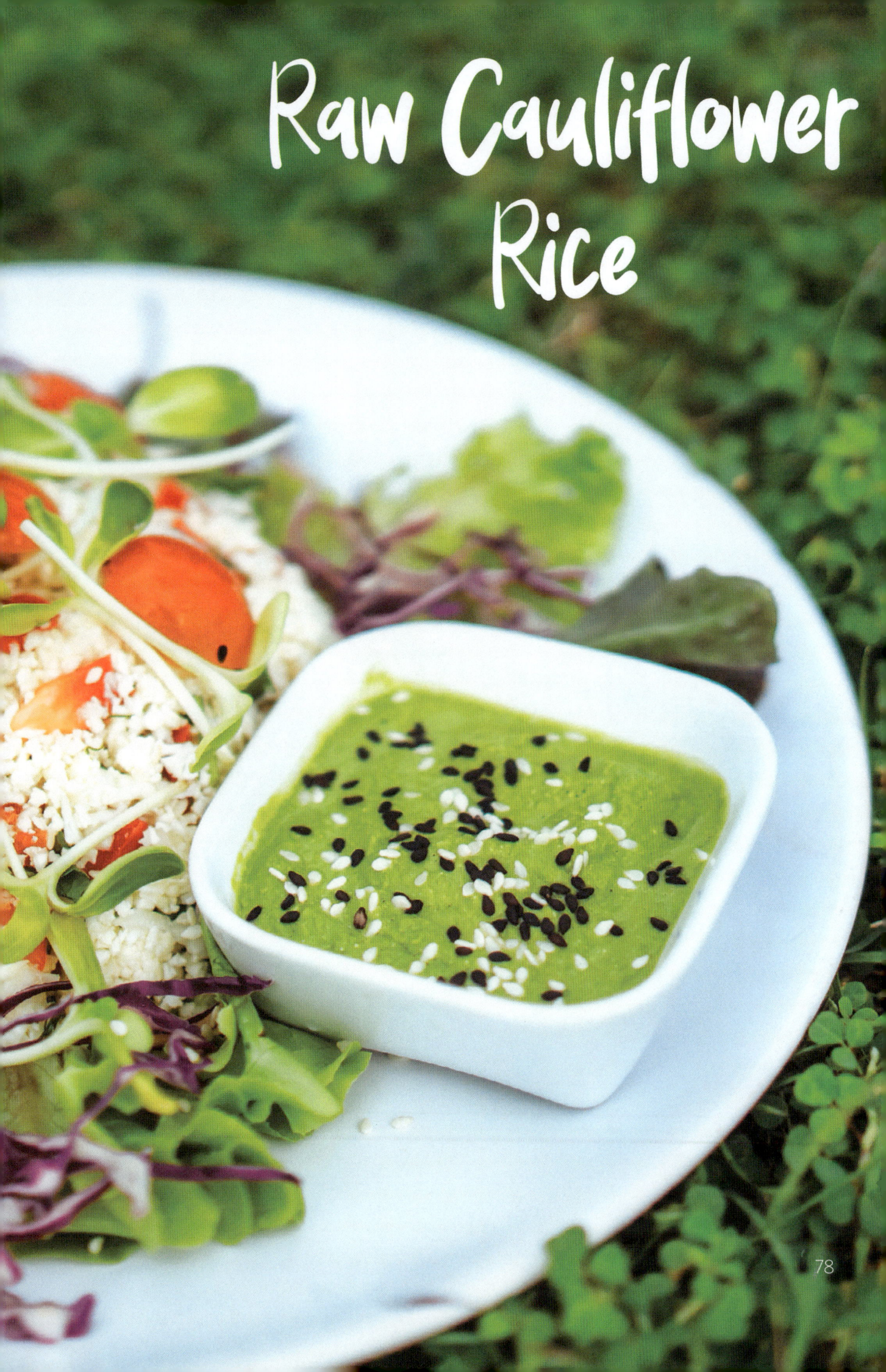

Raw Cucumber & Spirulina Soup

A light, clean bite and satisfying slurp. This chilled soup is a perfect starter food after a fast or belly-cleanse, or to uplift a tired heart and refresh after long day. Zesty Kale Pesto and fresh basil infuse with flavour and fragrance, while ginger adds a spicy kick. Top with fresh shavings of ginger and a single basil leaf for pretty presentation. Savour this one slowly.

INGREDIENTS

450 gr Cucumber, cold and peeled

5 – 6 Basil leaves

½ tsp Himalayan salt

1 tbsp Kale pesto (Page 123)

1 tsp Spirulina

5 gr Fresh ginger

INSTRUCTIONS

Put the first five ingredients and 3 grams of the ginger in a high-speed blender and blend until smooth. Ensure you use a cold cucumber (from the fridge)! Garnish with the remaining 2 grams of freshly grated ginger.

Serving Size: 1
Preparation Time: 15 minutes

Raw Gazpacho

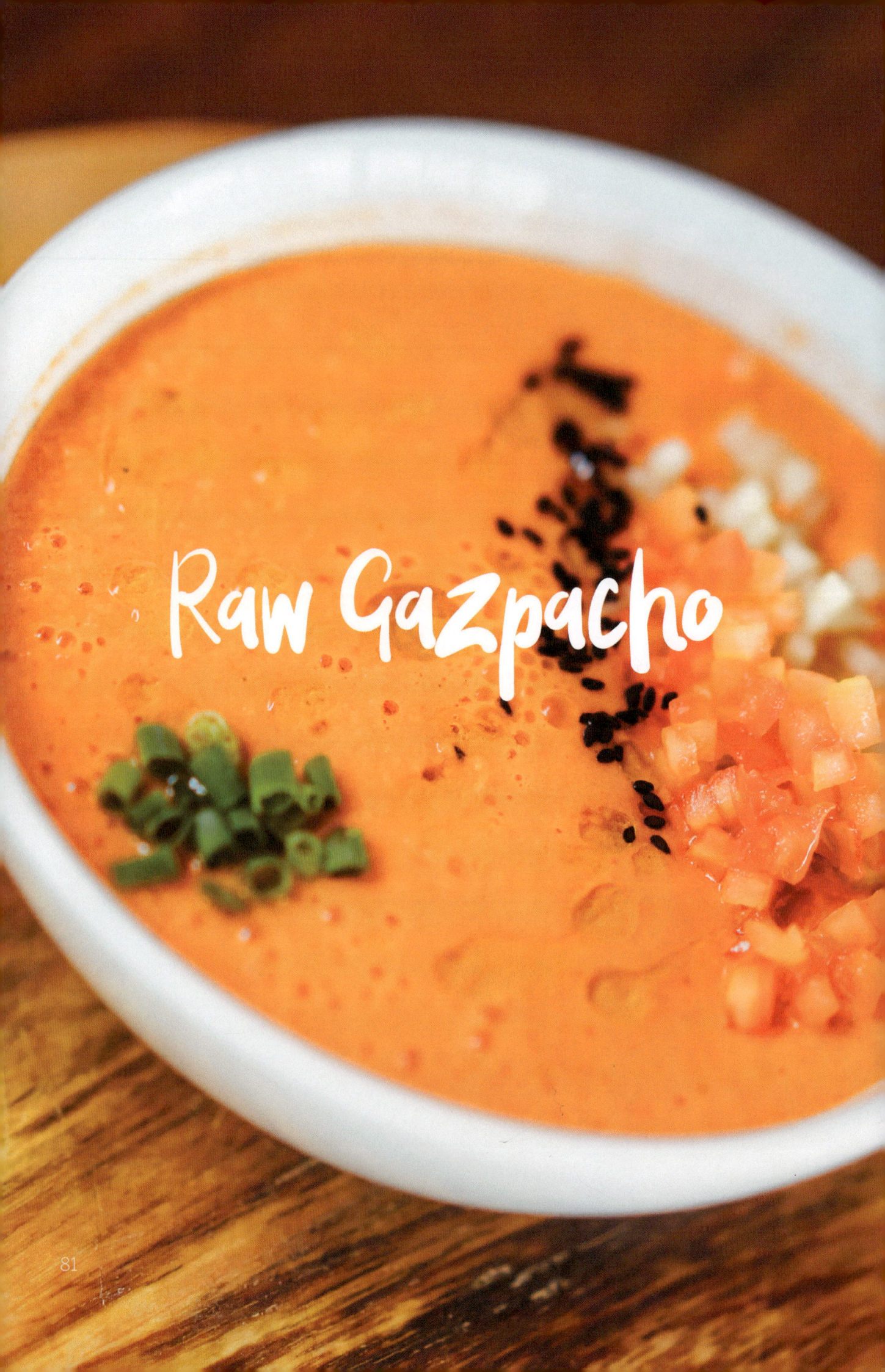

Punchy and pungent, flavour is abundant in this frothy favourite among Españoles, and everyone else in the world. Nutritious nightshady tomatoes and red capsicum join flavourful garlic and onion in this luscious, lip-smacking soup. Arouse the tongue's hidden desires with a first spoonful of this fragrant, light puree.

INGREDIENTS

1 Red bell pepper (approx. 200 gr)

1 Tomato (approx. 100 gr)

100 gr Cucumber

½ Clove of garlic

15 gr Red onion

½ tsp Himalayan salt

Pinch of Black pepper

1 tbsp Olive oil

Garnish: Chopped cucumber, tomato, and parsley.

INSTRUCTIONS

Put all ingredients in a high-speed blender and blend until the soup takes on a rustic consistency. Serve topped with tomato, cucumber, and parsley leaves, and a side of brown rice or quinoa.

Serving Size: 1
Preparation Time: 15 minutes

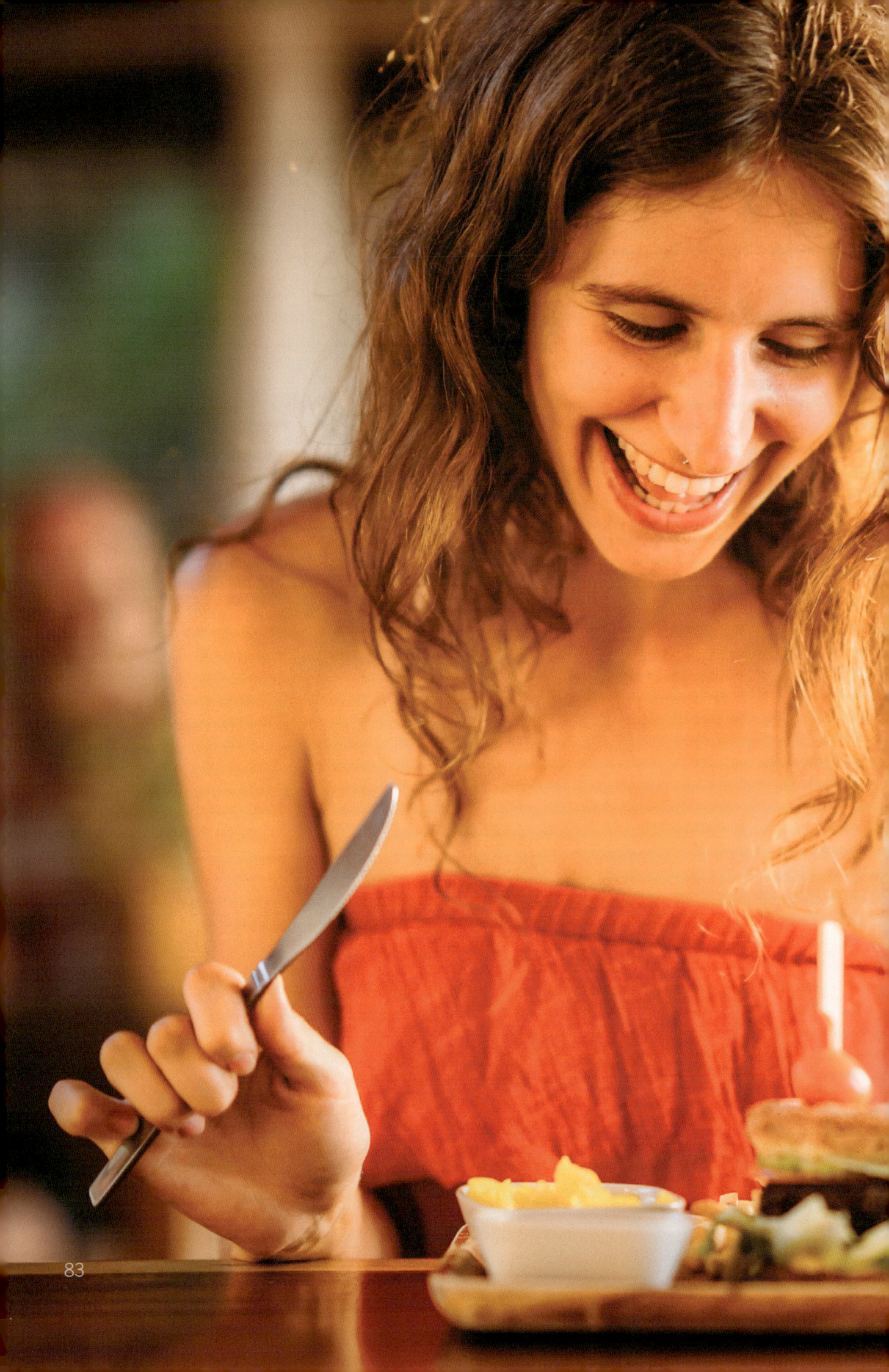

Main Dishes

This is pure sustenance. Meaty Roasted Chickpeas, smokey Baba Ganoush, and easy-breezy Tomato Salsa capture the heart of this wholesome and satisfying bowl. An effortless joy goes into preparing this mélange of wild ancestral legumes and nutrient-rich nightshades. Cumin and paprika are baked into gently roasted chickpeas with just a splash of virgin olive oil. Baba Ganoush mashes grilled eggplant with creamy tahini and a good smack of garlic and heating spices. Simple Tomato Salsa with coriander refreshes and balances the bowl.

INGREDIENTS

Prepare the following recipes:
Baba Ganoush, Sweet Potato Fries, Tomato Salsa, and Roasted Chickpeas (**see Sauces & Sides**).

50 gr Asparagus or long beans

50 gr Mixed salad greens

1 tbs Sesame seeds

1 slice of Lime

Plating

Heap generous amounts of each dish onto a bed of choice green salad leaves, and top with gently steamed asparagus or long beans and sweet potato fries. Sprinkle sesame seeds and give a generous squeeze of lime to the whole mix. Dig in and enjoy a playful mash-up of sauce and structure.

Serving Size: 1
Preparation Time: 20 minutes

Bliss Bowl

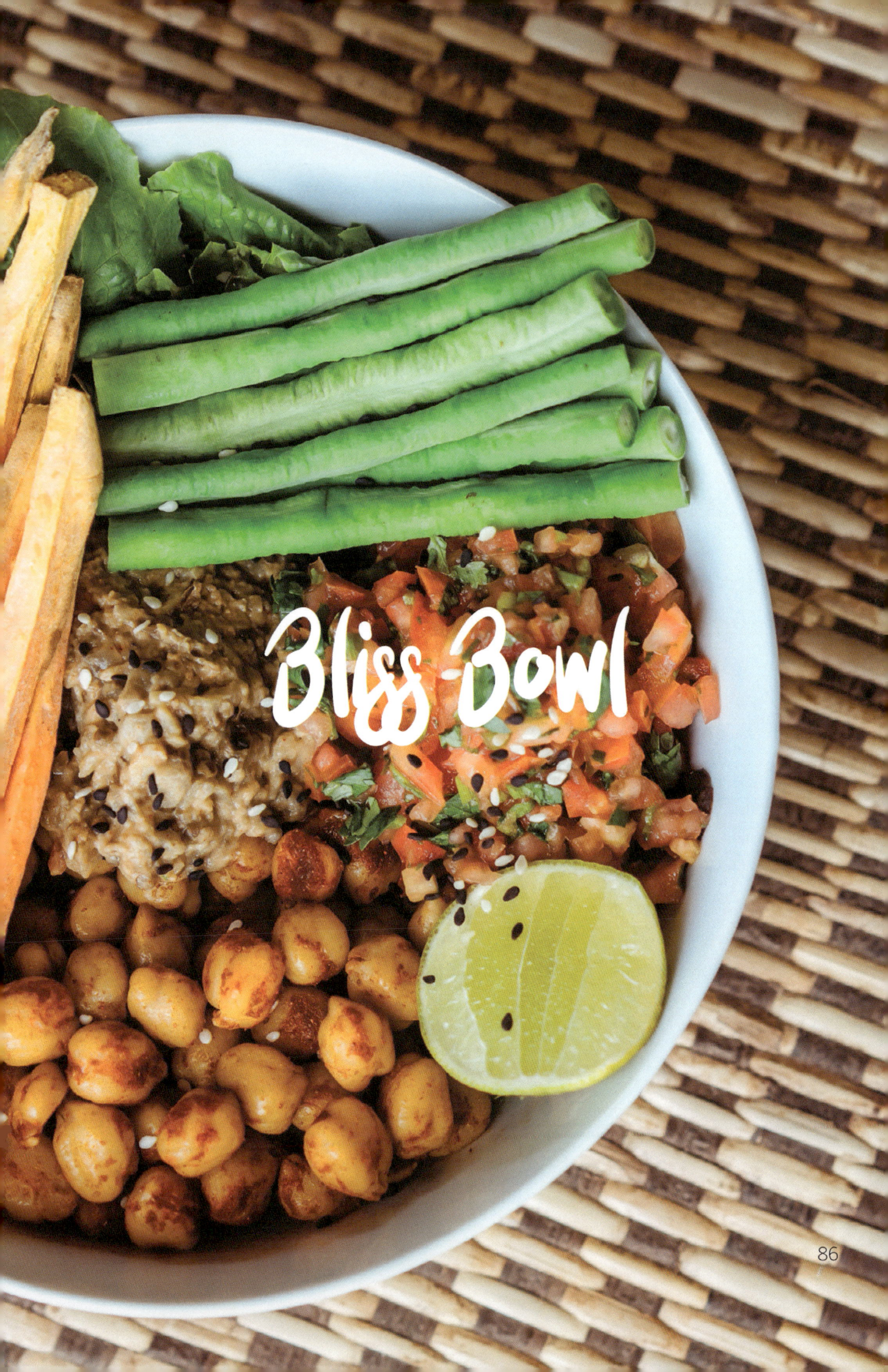

Nature's underground abundance features in this marvellous stack of plant-based bliss. Wild, voluptuous beetroots are grated and mixed with chopped walnuts, soy sauce, and chewy sun-dried tomatoes. Hints of smoked paprika and cinnamon coax your root essence into full submission. Smother with upgraded versions of classic tangy drippings, like Tomato Ketchup and Cashew Cheese, and deepen the delight with belly-warming Purple Sauerkraut, fermented with ginger and fresh coriander leaf. Bring the whole stack to a climax by adding fresh crisp lettuce, tomato, and sliced pickles.

INGREDIENTS

THE PATTY

150 gr Walnuts

2 tbsp Olive oil

1 clove Garlic, crushed

30 gr Onion, finely chopped

300 gr Raw beetroot, peeled and grated

2 tbsp Sun-dried tomatoes, finely chopped

¾ cup Water (more if needed)

2 tbsp Soy sauce

80 gr Almond powder

1 tsp Smoked paprika

Pinch of Ground cinnamon

INSTRUCTIONS

Blend the walnuts into a fine powder. Gently heat olive oil in a large frying pan, add crushed garlic and chopped onions and fry for about 2 minutes.

Add the beetroot, sun-dried tomatoes, and some water, and stir about 10 minutes, until soft. Transfer the mixture into a food processor and blend until smooth.

Add the prepared walnut powder, soy sauce, almond powder, paprika and cinnamon, and blend again. Divide the batter into four and shape each into a patty. Fry 2 – 3 minutes on each side until golden and crispy.

Plating

Charcoal buns add a delicious twist. Halve and toast, stacking your burger with layers of fresh salad, Tomato Ketchup (Page 125), Cashew Cheese (Page 128), Purple Sauerkraut (Page 129), and serve with Sweet Potato Fries (Page 116).

Serving Size: 4
Preparation Time: 15 minutes

Beetroot Burger

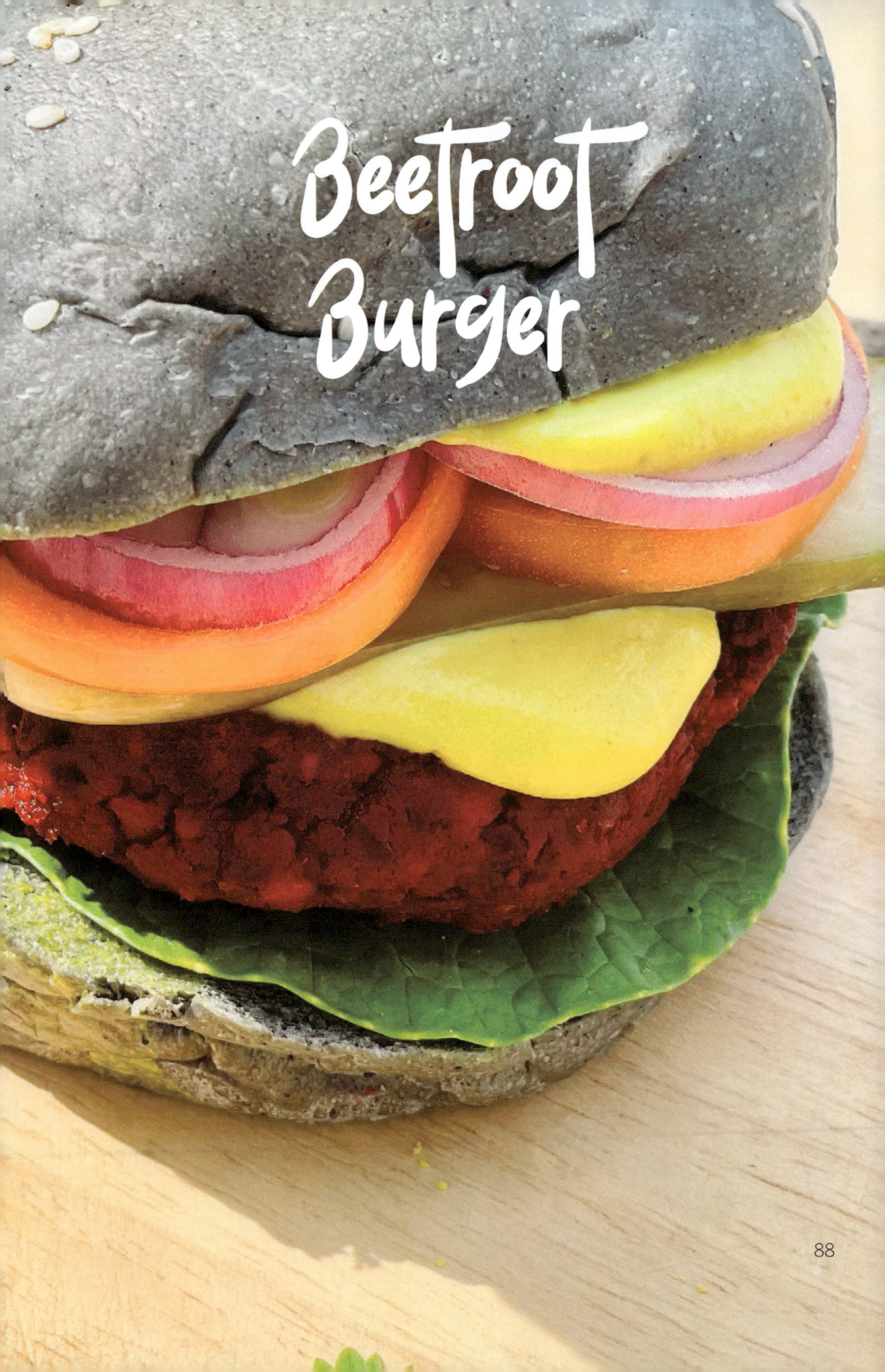

Om Ramen

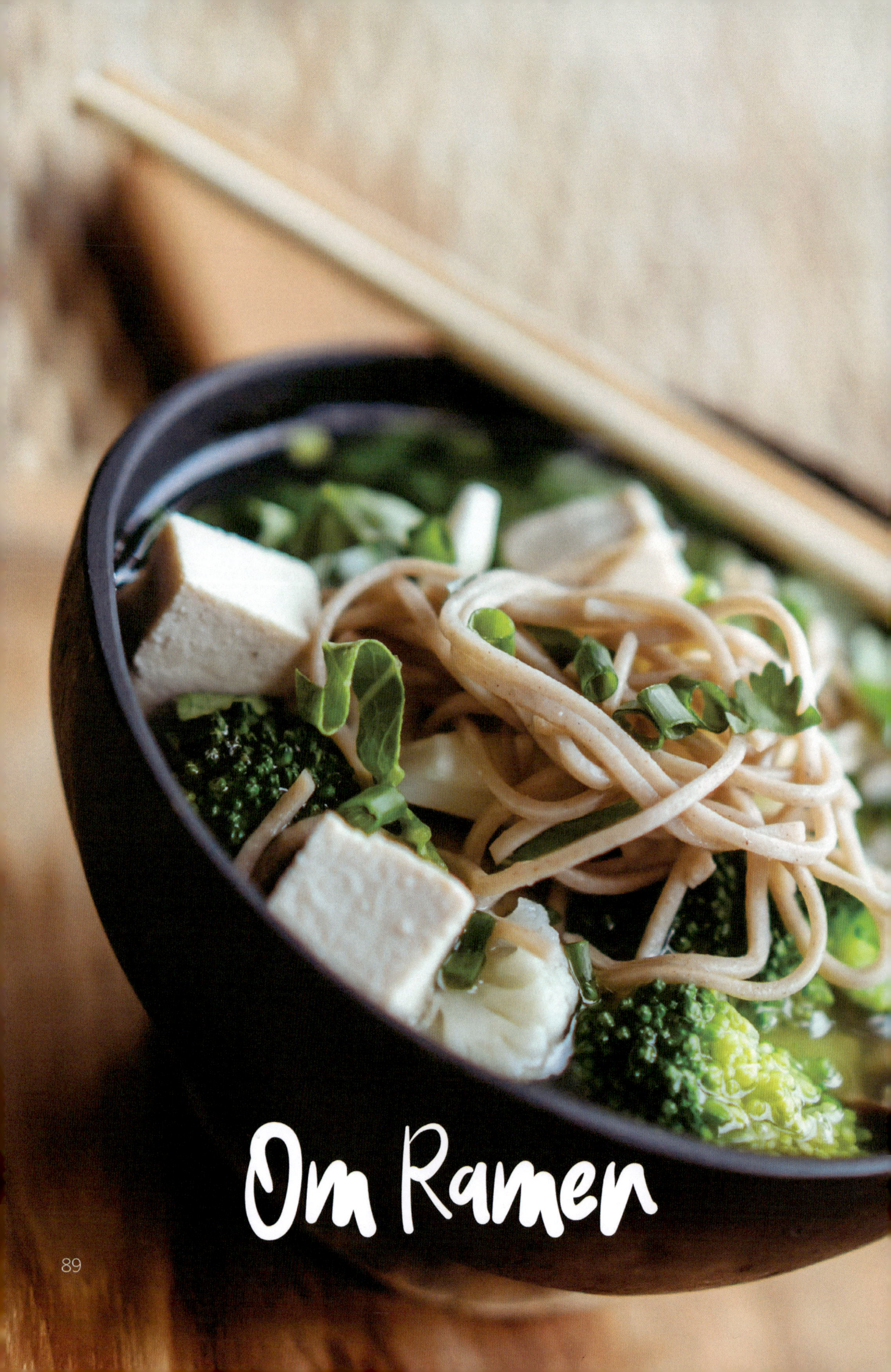

A classic miso-based noodle soup that's slurpy, satisfying, and delightfully textured. This Om-inspired ramen bowl is infused with fresh earthy flavour. Starting with a light and tangy fermented vegetable broth, chewy shiitake and fibre-rich cauliflower are added to create heartiness and texture. The vibrant green of lovingly wilted kale leaf expands the heart chakra. Born from the earth, kale is one of the few iron-rich foods that, when cooked, has an airy quality. Tender tofu slices and slender buckwheat noodles add structure and playfulness. Garnish with fresh spring onion, fragrant coriander leaf and sesame seeds. Savour this blissful bowl of wholesome goodness down to its last drop.

INGREDIENTS

1 tbsp Sesame oil	70 gr Cauliflower, (chopped into small florets)
½ tsp Chopped garlic	40 gr Kale leaf, cut into small slices
½ tsp Chopped ginger	40 gr Tofu
4 tbsp Chopped spring onions	100 gr Buckwheat noodles (pre-cooked)
2½ cups Vegetable broth	1 tbsp Coriander leaf, finely chopped
1 tbsp Miso paste	1 tsp Sesame seeds
30 gr Shiitake mushrooms, chopped	

INSTRUCTIONS

Heat sesame oil in a large pot on high for about 2 minutes until hot and simmering, but not smoking. Immediately toss in the garlic, ginger, and 2 tbsp spring onions. The onions will sizzle, turn bright green, and wilt almost immediately. Add the vegetable broth (you may substitute with regular water). Once warm, add the miso paste and whisk until combined. Add chopped mushrooms and cauliflower and cook for about 5 minutes. Toss in the kale leaf, tofu, and buckwheat noodles. Pour the soup into a bowl and serve with freshly chopped remaining spring onions, coriander and sesame seeds.

Serving Size: 1
Preparation Time: 15 minutes

Dal Tadka

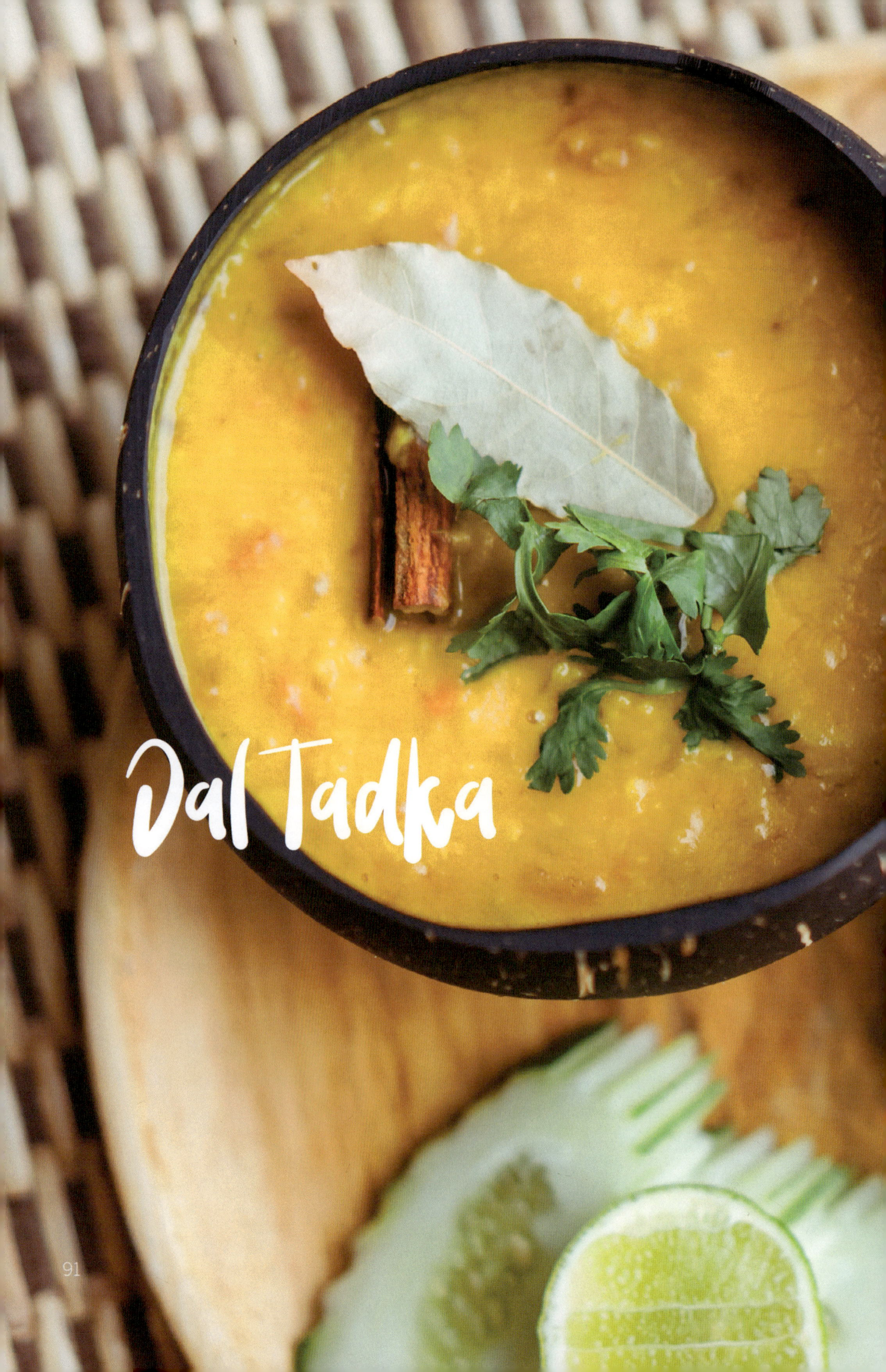

*A true belly warmer, manipura amplifier, and a most satisfying protein hit.
This traditional Indian stew is a crowd-pleaser that gives a healthy
dose of fiber, micronutrients, and most importantly, taste.
All the best Indian spices mingle here, seducing lentils with colour and flavour.
This dal is from no ordinary world. Pair with basmati rice and get all
nine essential amino acids in one delicious dish.*

INGREDIENTS

100 gr Moong dal (or yellow lentils)

2 tsp Turmeric powder

3 tbsp Rice oil

1 tsp Cumin seeds

2 – 3 Bay leaves

1 Small cinnamon stick

1 Small piece of ginger, finely chopped

1 Clove of garlic, finely chopped

1 Small green chilli pepper

100 gr Red onion, finely chopped

100 gr Tomatoes, finely chopped

1 tsp Himalayan salt

1 tbsp Coriander, finely chopped

INSTRUCTIONS

Soak the moong dal or lentils for one hour. Then, rinse thoroughly and put them in a pot with a pinch of salt and 1 tsp of turmeric powder, and boil for about 30 minutes. Heat the oil together with cumin seeds, bay leaves, cinnamon stick, ginger, garlic, and green chilli pepper. Fry until the garlic and ginger become slightly brown, then add the chopped onion and cook for an additional 5 minutes. Add the tomatoes, salt, and remaining turmeric powder and fry for about 2 minutes. Add the lentils and allow to simmer for another 5 minutes until they reach the desired consistency. Transfer the dal into a bowl, and serve with freshly chopped coriander leaves and a side of basmati rice or quinoa.

Serving Size: 1
Preparation Time: 90 minutes

Drown your taste buds in this belly-warming, mouthwatering explosion of flavour from the Far East. The aroma might be your most passionate encounter with food, but just wait until you taste it! Spicy curry paste tests the tongue's limits with a brazen heat that commands attention. Rustic pumpkin, sweet potato, and turmeric dwell in rich, velvety coconut milk and arouse sensuality, creative magic, and a warm feeling of home. A hint of sweet balances the spice and lures you in for more. Serve with cooling kaffir leaf garnish and wholesome brown rice.

INGREDIENTS

1½ cups Coconut milk

½ tbsp Coconut curry paste

1 tsp Himalayan salt

Pinch of Turmeric powder

⅓ tbsp Coconut sugar paste

100 gr Sweet potato, chopped into bite-size cubes

100 gr Pumpkin, chopped into bite-size cubes

10 gr Kaffir leaves, finely sliced

INSTRUCTIONS

Heat the coconut milk in a large pot and add the curry paste, salt, turmeric and coconut sugar paste. Cook for about 2 minutes then add the sweet potato and pumpkin. Cook for 10 more minutes until the vegetables are tender. Serve with sliced kaffir leaves on top and a side of brown rice or quinoa.

Serving Size: 1
Preparation Time: 30 minutes

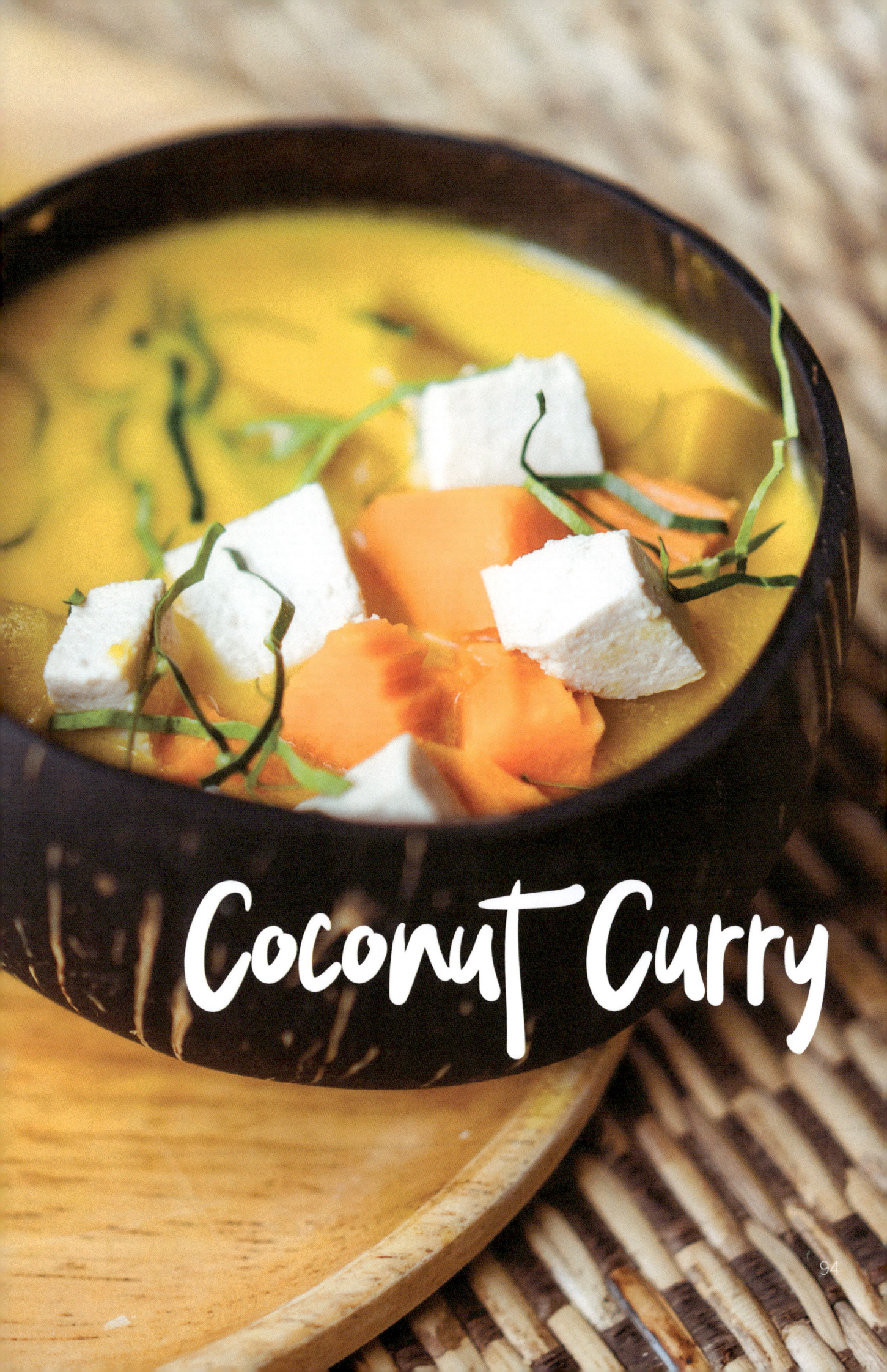

Coconut Curry

Spicy Meaty Mushrooms

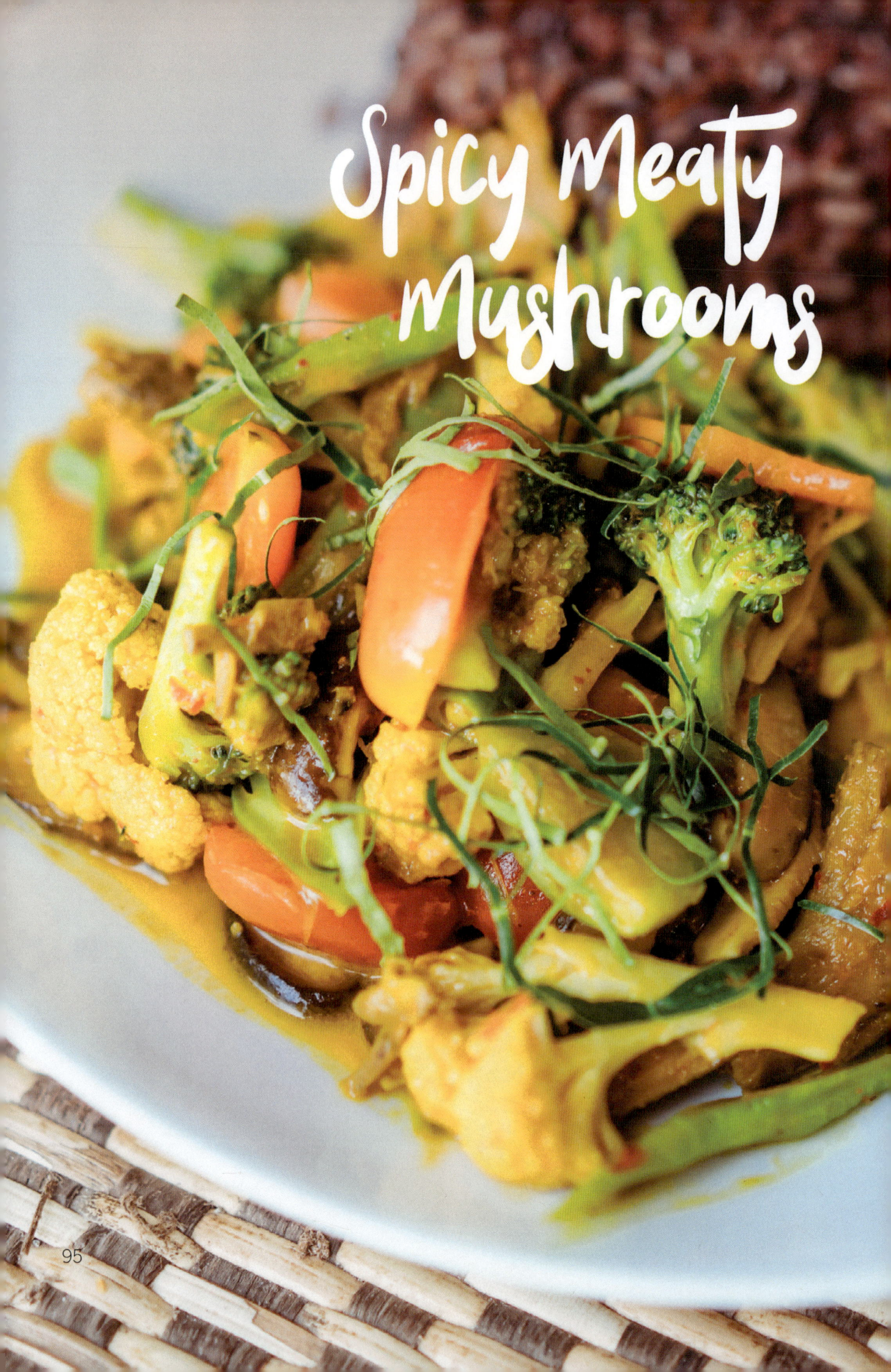

This is where all the fun is. A teasing tango of texture, taste, spice, and earthy bliss. Both fresh and fermented mushrooms offer a taste of the wild and primordial underground ~ a spirit released with the addition of creamy coconut milk, garden vegetables, and fragrant herbs. One bite leads to another, which leads to another, until you surrender to the intuitive pleasure of eating real, wholesome food. You'll want this one to go on forever.

INGREDIENTS

- 2 tbsp Rice oil
- ½ tbsp Panang curry paste
- ½ cup Coconut milk
- Pinch of Turmeric powder
- ½ tbsp Coconut sugar paste
- 40 gr Cauliflower, chopped into florets
- 30 gr Broccoli, chopped into florets
- 15 gr Small green eggplants, chopped into bite-size cubes
- 15 gr Long snakebean, or 4 green beans, cut into 4 inch pieces
- 1 Small carrot, chopped into bite-size cubes
- 50 gr Fresh shiitake mushrooms, sliced
- 25 gr Fermented mushrooms
- 2 tbsp Mushroom soy sauce
- 1 Small tomato, cut into 4 pieces
- 7 - 8 Basil leaves
- 5 - 6 Kaffir lime leaves

INSTRUCTIONS

In a large pan, heat the rice oil and panang curry paste on medium heat for only a few seconds to prevent burning. Then add the coconut milk, turmeric, and coconut sugar paste, and cook for approximately 1 minute. Add the cauliflower, broccoli, green eggplant, long bean, carrot, fresh mushrooms, fermented mushrooms, and soy sauce. Simmer for about 5 minutes, then add the tomato, basil leaves, and kaffir lime leaves. Serve with a side of brown rice or quinoa.

Serving Size: 1
Preparation Time: 15 minutes

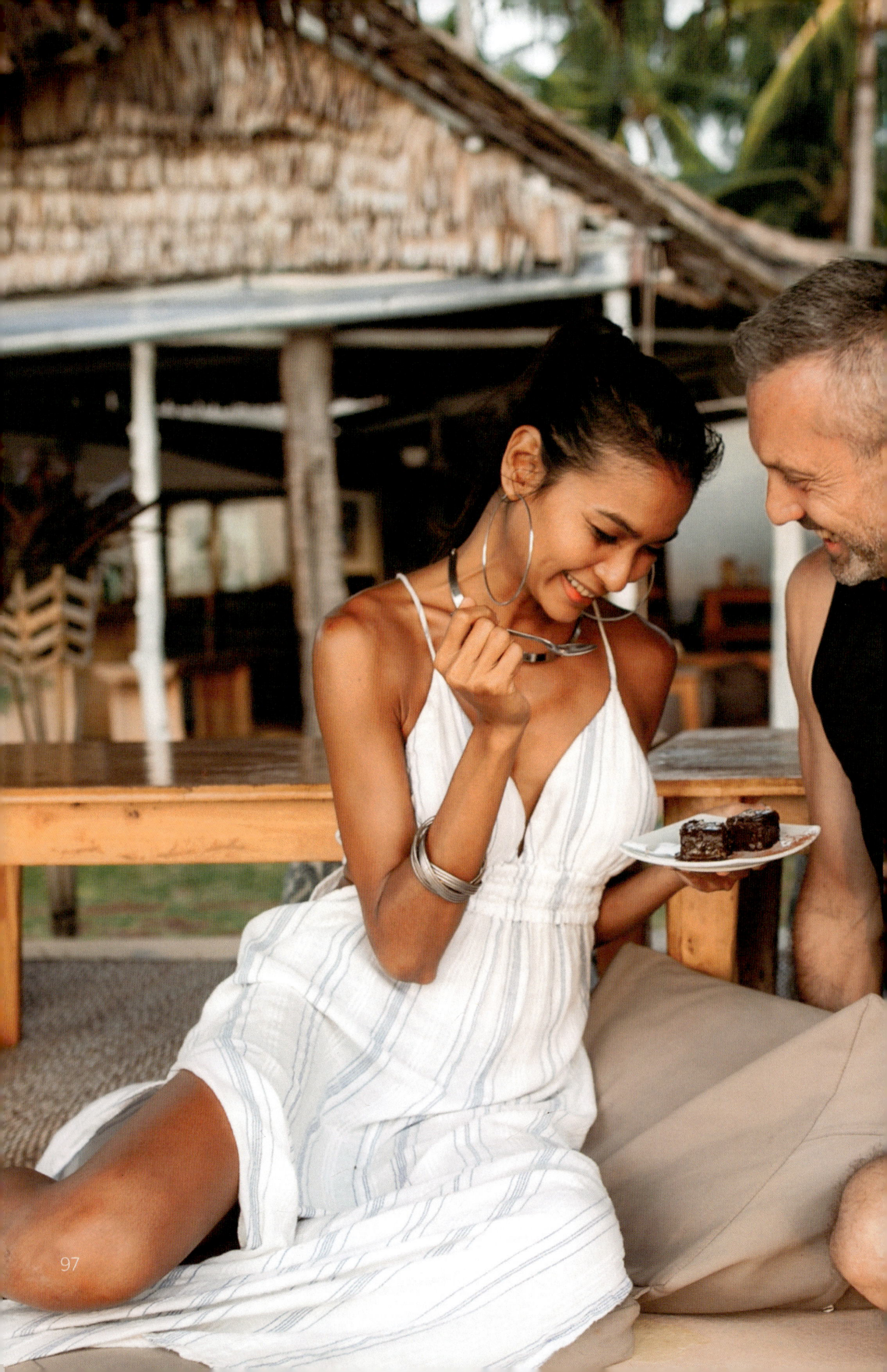

Desserts

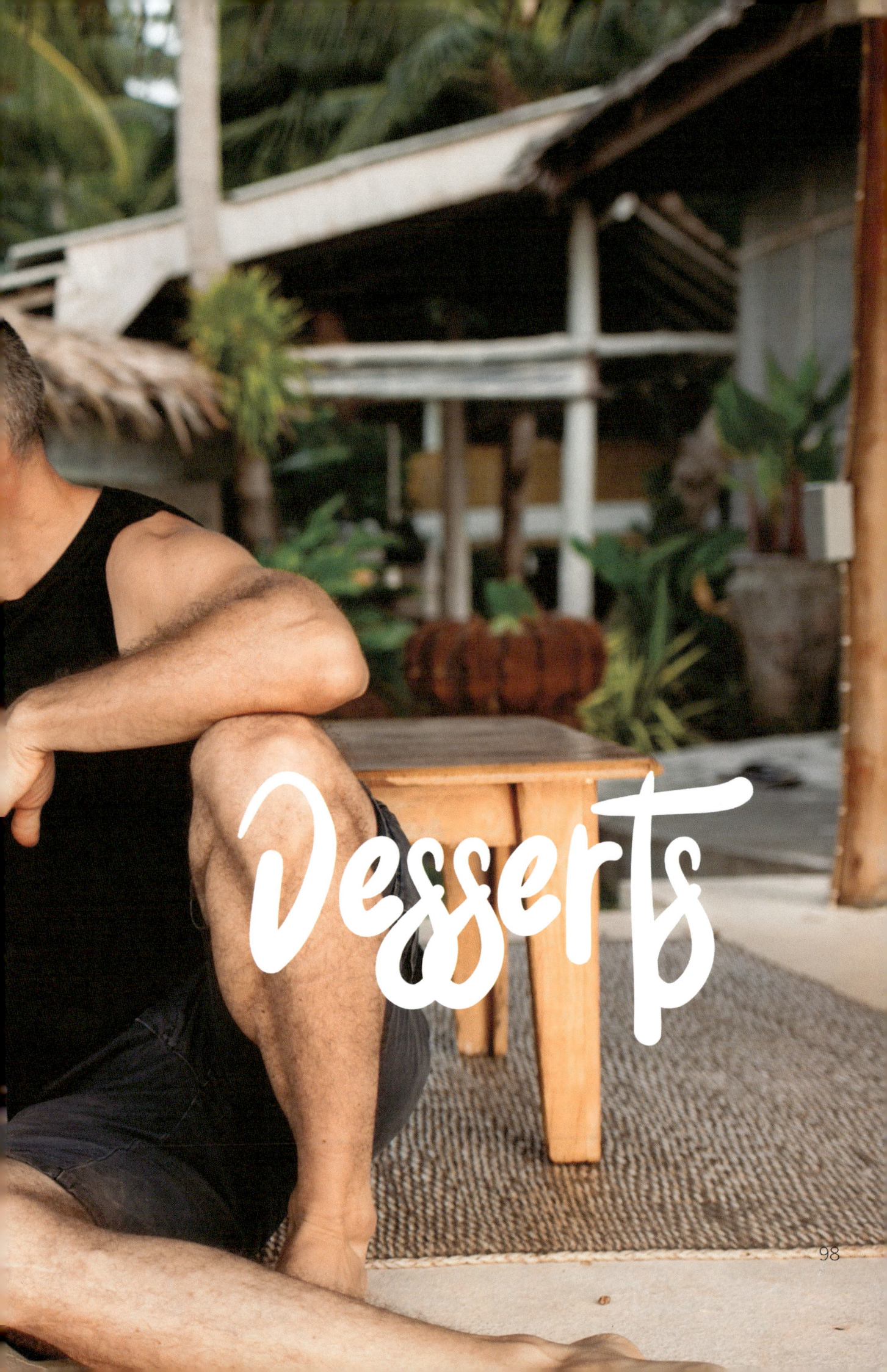

Raw Cheesecake

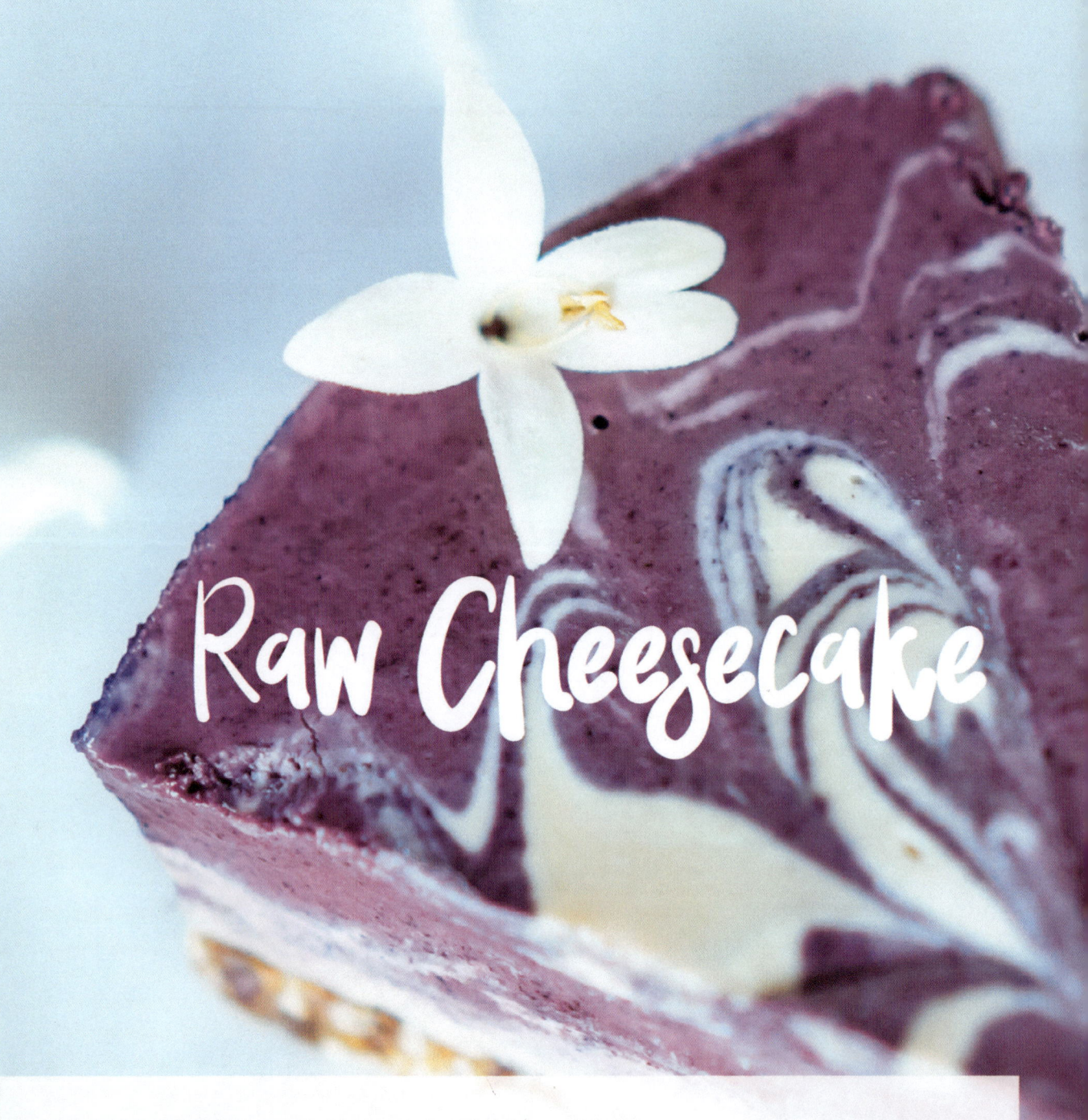

A wedge of the Divine. Dense raw cheesecake satisfies your craving for innocent indulgence with three layers of sweet and nutty nom nom. Deep dark cacao meets banana, a most cosmic match and mood enhancer, stacked regally upon a chewy and delightfully unadorned date-nut base. Coconut gifts its subtle sweetness and superfood fatty goodness throughout. A hint of vanilla teases the intuition. Take just a moment or two of sensual stillness before you plunge into this raw sensation.

INGREDIENTS

1ST LAYER
300 gr Almonds
250 gr Dates

2ND LAYER
400 gr Cashew nuts (soaked 6 hours)
⅔ cup Coconut oil
⅔ cup Coconut flower syrup
1 tsp Vanilla essence

3RD LAYER
100 gr Cashew nuts
⅔ cup Coconut oil
⅔ cup Coconut flower syrup
1 tsp Vanilla essence
8 tbsp Cacao powder
6 Ripe bananas

INSTRUCTIONS

For the 1st layer:
Blend the almonds and dates together in a food processor. Pulse to achieve a sticky mixture, then press evenly into an 8-inch round cake mold lined with parchment paper.

For the 2nd layer:
Submerge cashew nuts in lukewarm water in a large bowl and soak for 6 hours. Strain the cashew nuts and put them in a high-speed blender with coconut oil, coconut syrup, and vanilla. Blend until the mixture is smooth and creamy. Gently pour on top the almond base. Spread evenly.

For the 3rd layer:
Combine cashew nuts, coconut oil, coconut syrup, vanilla, cacao powder and banana in the blender and pulse into a puree. Pour on top of the second cashew cream layer to completely cover the cake. Freeze for 8 hours or overnight.

To serve, allow the cake to sit at room temperature for 15 minutes to soften just enough so a knife can glide through.

Serving Size: 12
Preparation Time: 1 day

Raw Chocolate Fudge

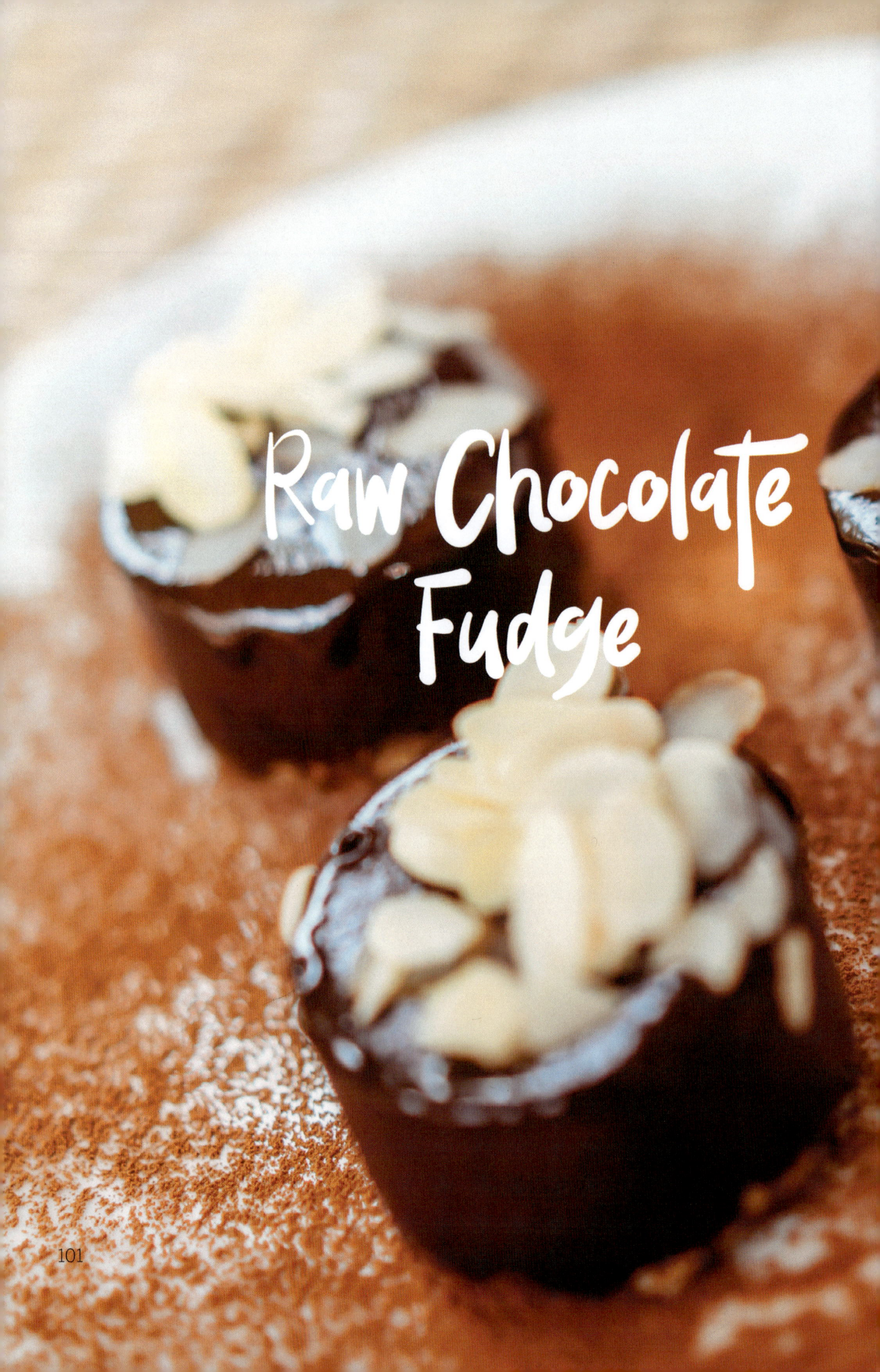

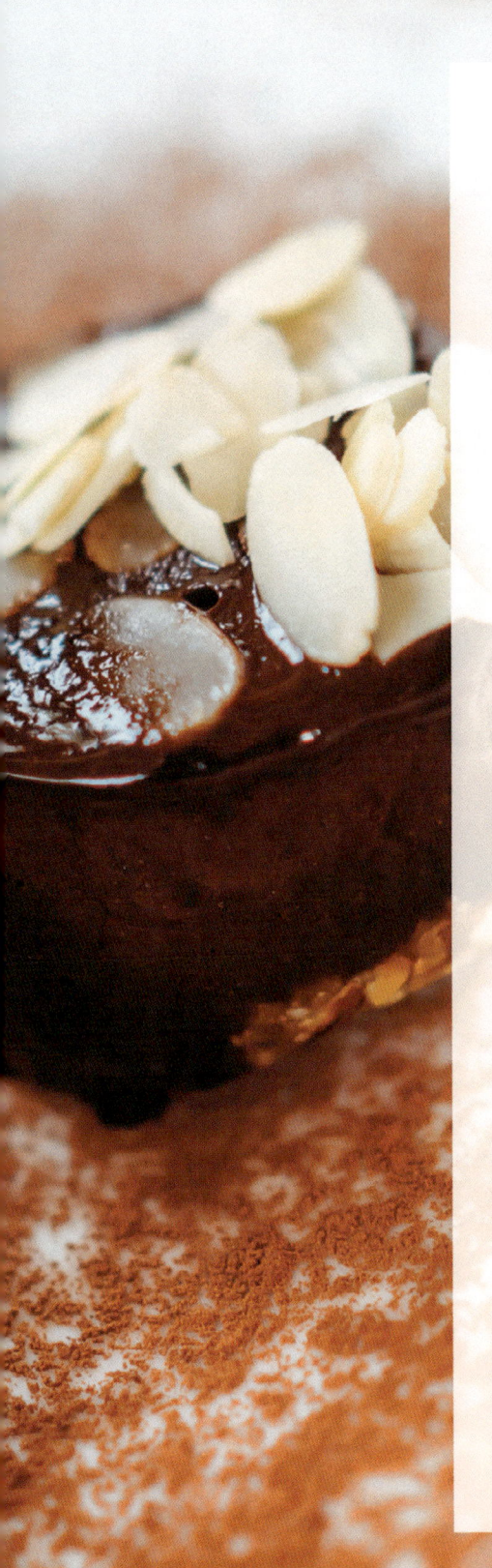

*Three raw superfoods deliver a seductive encounter with chocolate that is exquisitely simple, surprisingly rare. Each two-bite mound is sculpted and chilled into perfect form until it meets your tongue, where it surrenders into a melty, mouthwatering glimpse of heaven.
Keep chilled for a more rapturous experience.*

INGREDIENTS

10 tbsp Raw cacao powder
1 cup Coconut flower syrup
⅔ cup Coconut oil
1 cup Slithered almonds
(For this recipe, you'll need a 12 portion silicone chocolate mold)

INSTRUCTIONS

Whisk together all ingredients in a large bowl until the chocolate cream is completely smooth. Transfer the mixture to the silicone mold and spread evenly. Refrigerate for a minimum of 4 hours.

Serving Size: 12
Preparation Time: 5 hours

Raw Snickers Bar

If heaven is a snack, this is it. Rich and chocolatey, nutty and chewy ~ all the natural bounty of the tropics come together to form this cosmic rockstar. Grounded with crushed peanuts, layered with coconut-infused caramel, and lifted by raw cacao powder. Dive into this delectable dessert bar with two ambitious bites or nibble at a slow, sensual pace.

INGREDIENTS

BASE	CARAMEL LAYER	DIPPING CHOCOLATE
1 kg Raw peanuts	400 gr Dates	½ cup Coconut flower syrup
300 gr Dates	400 gr Coconut syrup	½ cup Coconut oil
4 tbsp Coconut oil	5 tbsp Carob powder	4 tbsp Cacao powder
4 tbsp Coconut flower syrup	⅔ cup Coconut oil	

INSTRUCTIONS

Preheat the oven to 180°C. Arrange the peanuts on a baking tray and roast, tossing occasionally, until they are almost done. Allow them to cool for 10 minutes before proceeding.

For the base:
Pulse the peanuts into small pieces in a high-power food processor, add the dates, coconut oil and coconut syrup, and blend to a sticky dough. Press the dough into a square tray lined with parchment paper and store in the freezer.

For the caramel:
Blend the dates, coconut syrup, carob powder and coconut oil until completely smooth. Using a spatula, spread the caramel evenly over the base, and return to freezer for 2 more hours until the base and caramel are firm.

Remove the frozen filling from the tray. Using a sharp knife, cut into bar-sized pieces and freeze while you make the dipping sauce.

For the dipping chocolate:
Combine the coconut syrup, coconut oil, and cacao powder in a large bowl. Remove the bars from the freezer and place them into the bowl of dipping chocolate, one at a time. Use two forks to flip each bar until completely coated. Carefully place the bars onto a plate lined with parchment paper, and allow them to cool in the fridge for 15 minutes, until the chocolate coating has completely hardened.

Serving Size: 32
Preparation Time: 5 hours

Mint Cupcake

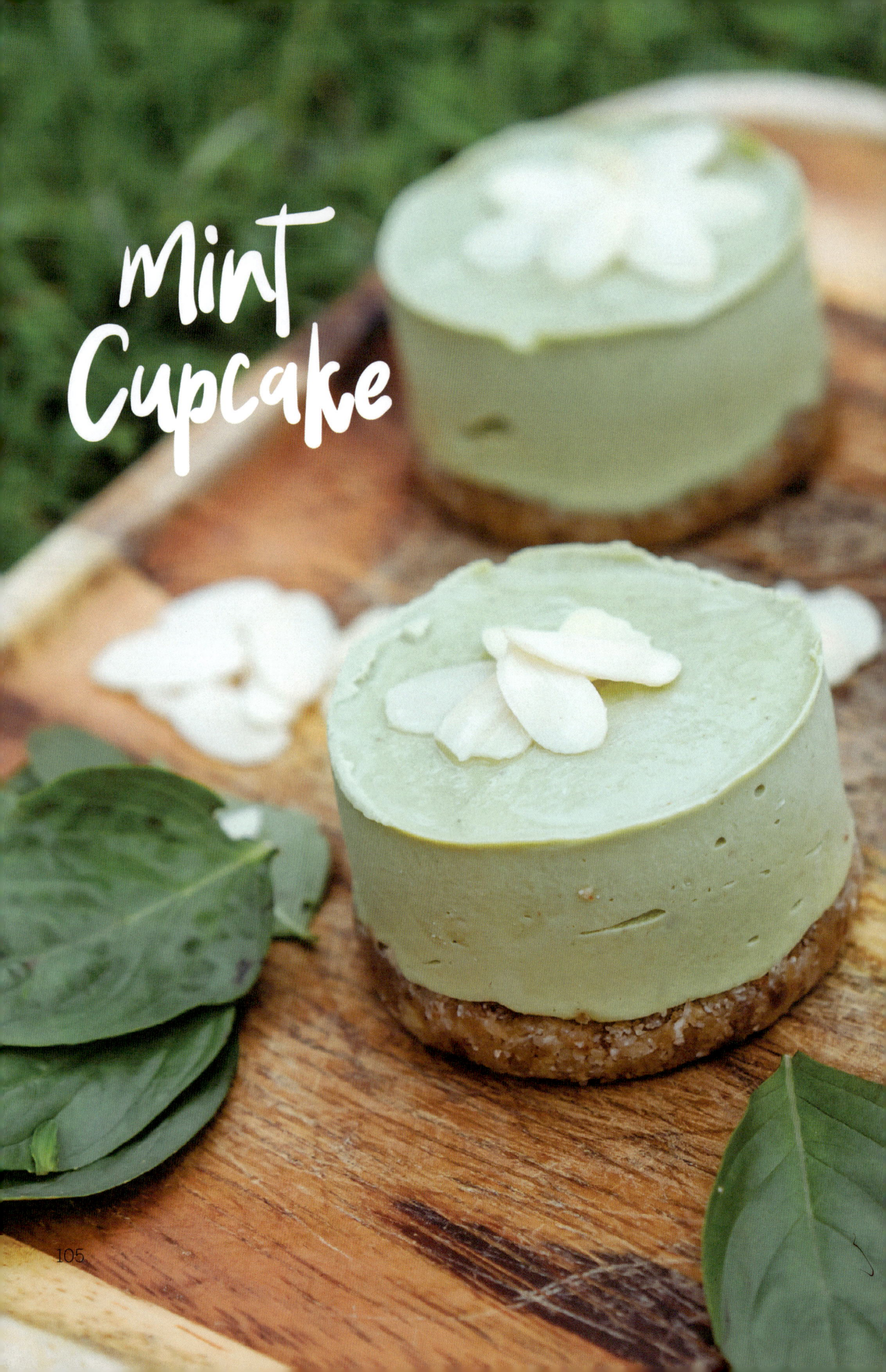

The food of the Gods meets mint in a cup of velvety loving joy. This one's worth the effort. Packed with a superfood punch, protein-rich spirulina hides with teasing, sensual flavors of coconut and mouth-cooling mint. The added wonders of dense, grounding nuts and earthly sweet dates form a chewy, satisfying base you might consider eating all on its own. But wait until you top it with sweet, minty magic!

INGREDIENTS

BASE

120 gr Almonds
150 gr Walnuts
120 gr Dates
1 tsp Cardamom
1 tbsp Tahini
Pinch of Himalayan salt

1ST LAYER

400 gr Soaked cashew nuts
2 tbsp Lime juice
½ cup Coconut syrup
½ cup Coconut oil
50 gr Fresh mint
Pinch of Himalayan salt
½ tsp Spirulina
2 tsp High-grade mint extract

INSTRUCTIONS

For the base:
Add almonds, walnuts, dates, cardamom, tahini, and salt in a food processor and pulse until well combined. Press the dough into an 8-cup silicone mold and store in the fridge while you prepare the filling.

For the 1st layer:
Blend all ingredients for the first layer of the filling in a high-speed blender until smooth. Take the silicone mold out of the freezer and add the puree on top of the chilled base, then freeze for at least 20 minutes.

Serving Size: 1 batch
Preparation Time: 3 hours

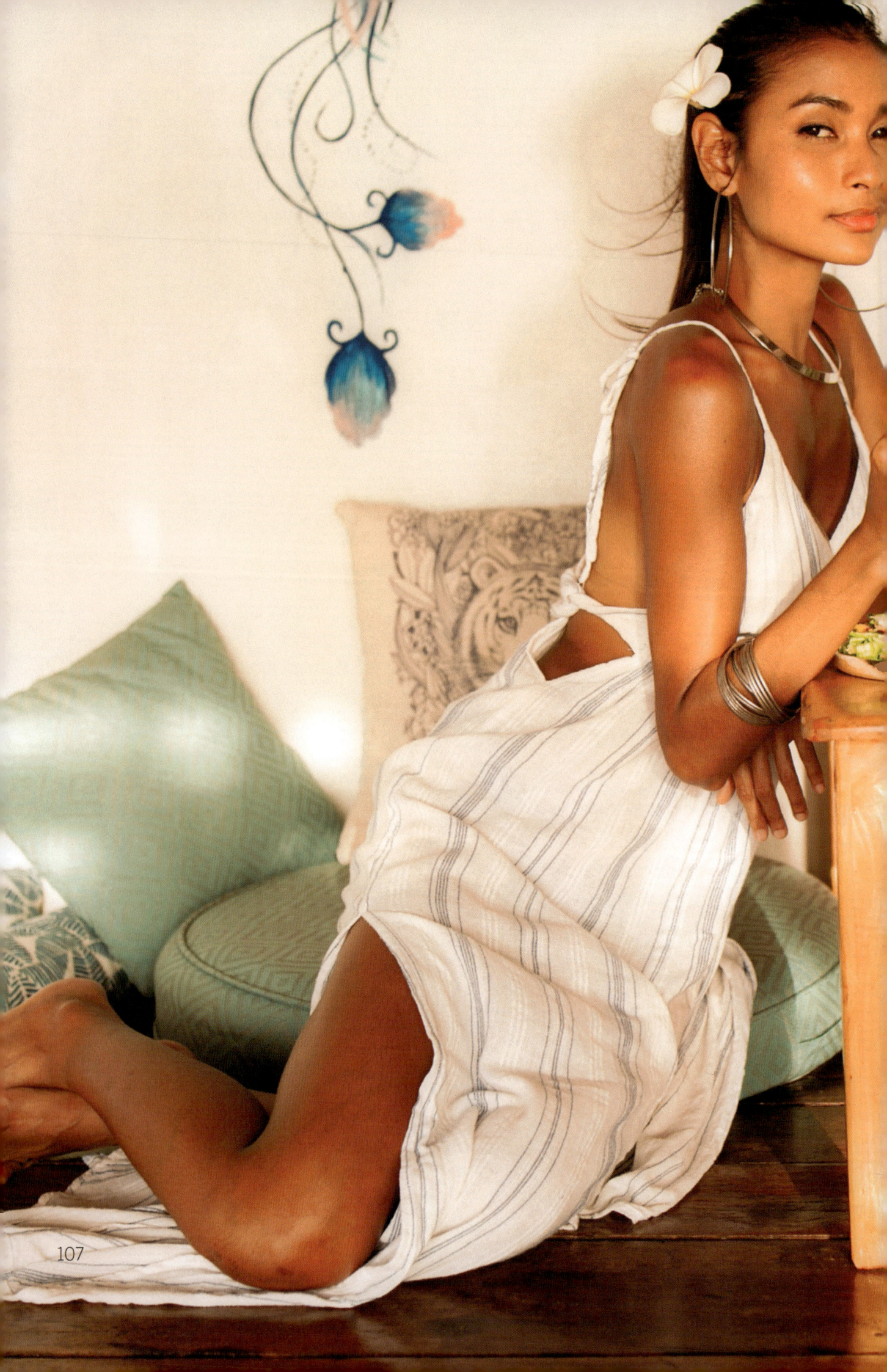

Sauces & Sides

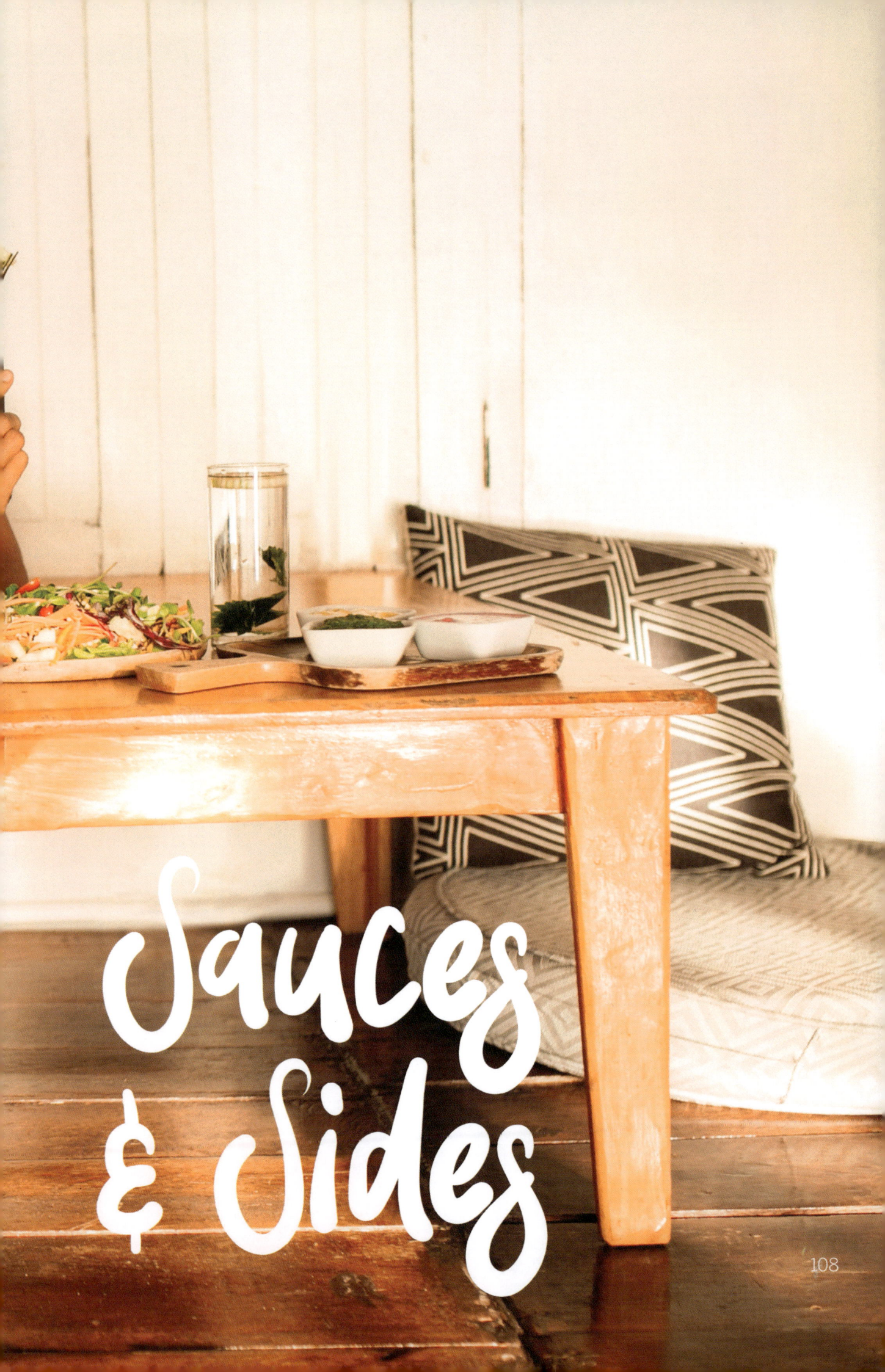

Orange Olive Oil Dressing

Simple and succulent, you'll want to drench every salad in this citrus sensation. Whisk well, serve generously, and allow time for these two flavours to merge with your favourite salad or pilaf.

INGREDIENTS

½ cup Freshly squeezed orange juice
2 tbsp Olive oil
Pinch of Himalayan salt

INSTRUCTIONS

Mix together all ingredients and pour generously over your salad.

Serving Size: 1
Preparation Time: 3 minute

Tomato Salsa

An invigorating kick of fresh juicy soul inhabits this chunky tomato salsa. Simple and scantily dressed for a natural taste. Use anywhere salsa lives, but especially atop the Bliss Bowl.

INGREDIENTS

150 gr Tomatoes
Pinch of Himalayan salt
1 tsp Coriander leaf, chopped
1 tsp Olive oil

INSTRUCTIONS

Chop the tomatoes into hearty chunks, combine with salt and chopped coriander. Drizzle with olive oil.

Serving Size: 1
Preparation Time: 5 minutes

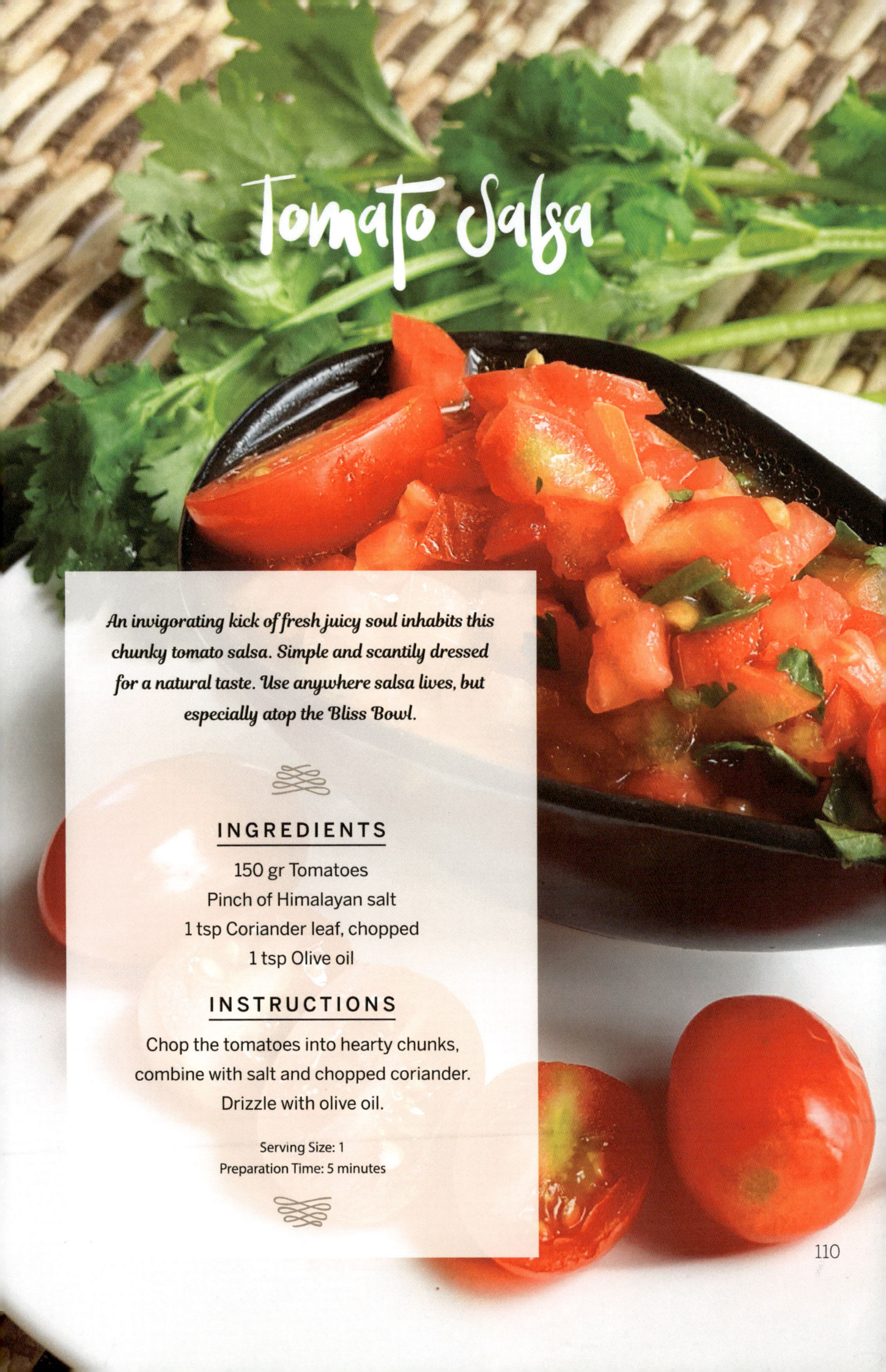

These snappy little omega-rich bites have an audible crunch and exceptional chew that will keep your belly happy and you coming back for more. Sensationally crisp and delicious, they side with any salad, soup, or serve as a simple snack.

INGREDIENTS

700 gr Carrots

60 gr Red onion

60 gr White onion

50 gr White sesame seeds

50 gr Sunflower seeds

50 gr Pumpkin seeds

50 gr Flax seeds

100 gr Flaxseed powder

½ tsp Himalayan salt

INSTRUCTIONS

Add the carrots and onion in a food processor and blend roughly, being careful not to overmix, transfer into a bowl. Add sesame seeds, sunflower seeds, pumpkin seeds, and flax seeds to the food processor, and blend again roughly. Then, combine both mixtures, and add the flaxseed powder and salt. Spread the mixture thinly onto dehydrator trays fitted with non-stick sheets, and pre-cut or mark the desired size for the crackers. Set the dehydrator to 45°C for about 16 hours. Then, peel the back to turn the crackers directly onto the dehydrator tray and dehydrate for an additional 4 hours, or until they are completely dry and crispy. Store the crackers in a dry and sealed container.

Serving Size: 1 batch
Preparation Time: 1 day

Raw Seeded Crackers

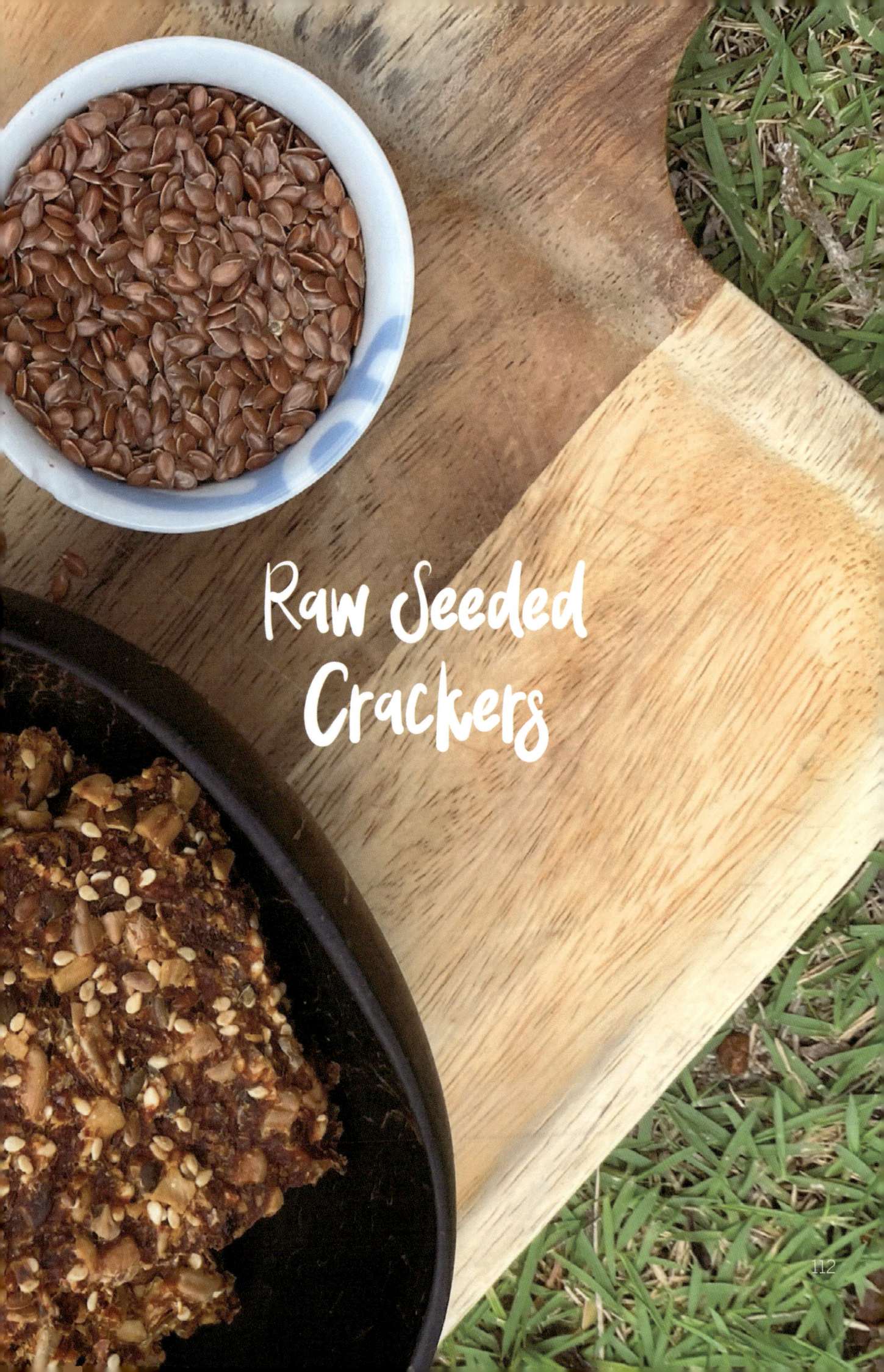

This nutrient-dense Levantine dip never tasted so good.
The secret? Fresh organic cumin and smoked paprika, high-quality olive oil, and hand-squeezed lime juice. And let's not forget the bliss of roasted eggplant mashed with freshly chopped garlic and rich, creamy tahini from whole sesame seeds. Innocently decadent enough to eat by the spoonful.

INGREDIENTS

1 kg Eggplant

5 tbsp Olive oil

100 gr Tahini

2 cloves of Garlic, chopped

½ tsp Himalayan salt

2 tbsp Lime juice

½ tsp Cumin powder

Pinch of Smoked paprika, for garnish

INSTRUCTIONS

Preheat the oven to 230°C. Halve the eggplants lengthwise and drizzle lightly with olive oil. Place them on a baking pan with the halved sides down. Roast for about 35-40 minutes, until the eggplants' interior is very tender. Allow to cool, then flip and scoop out the flesh with a large spoon. Using a large fork, mash the meat in a large bowl, then add tahini, chopped garlic, salt, lime juice, and cumin, and continue mashing until smooth. Dust with a pinch of smoked paprika.

Serving Size: 1 batch
Preparation Time: 1 hour

Baba Ganoush

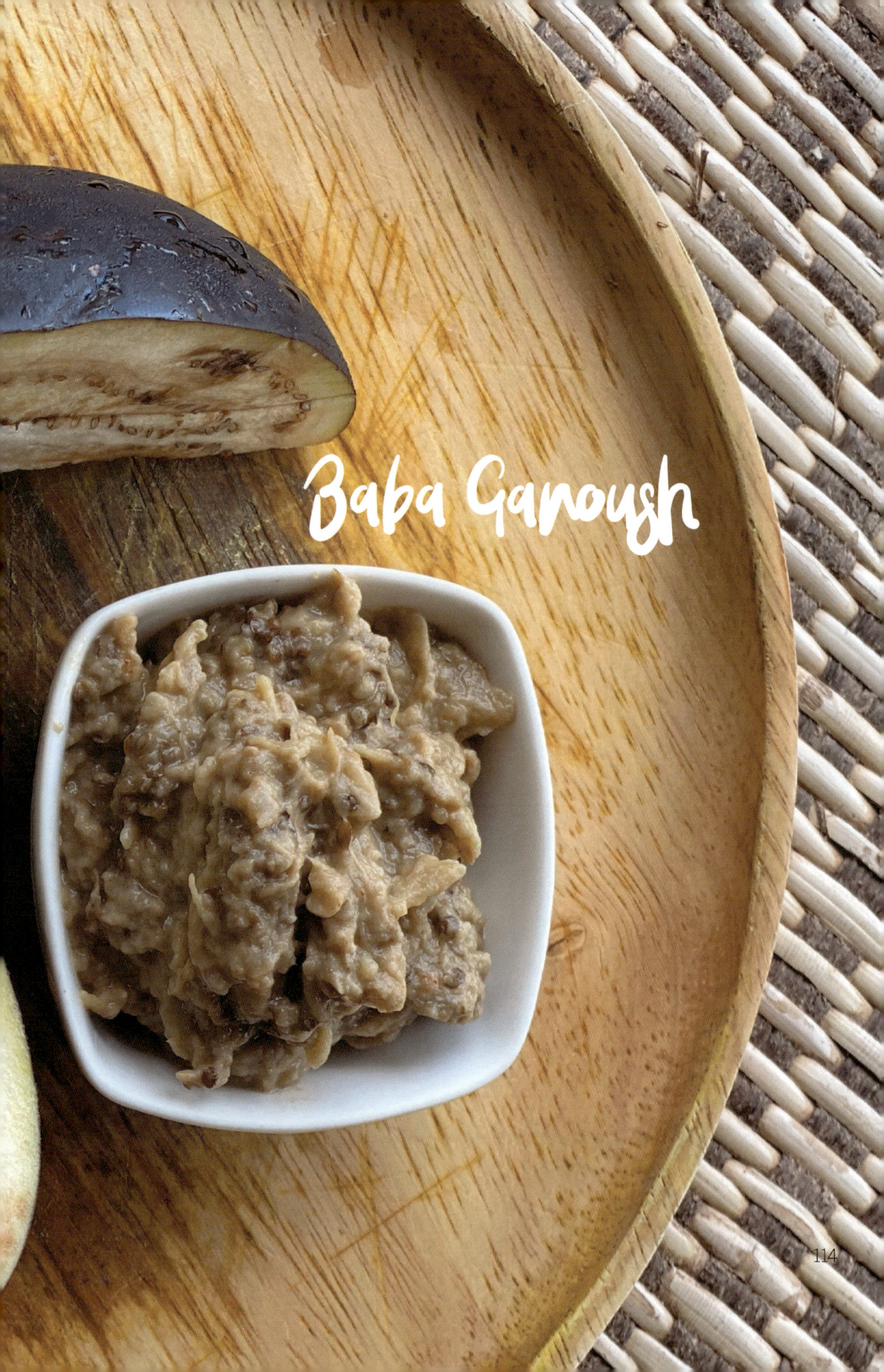

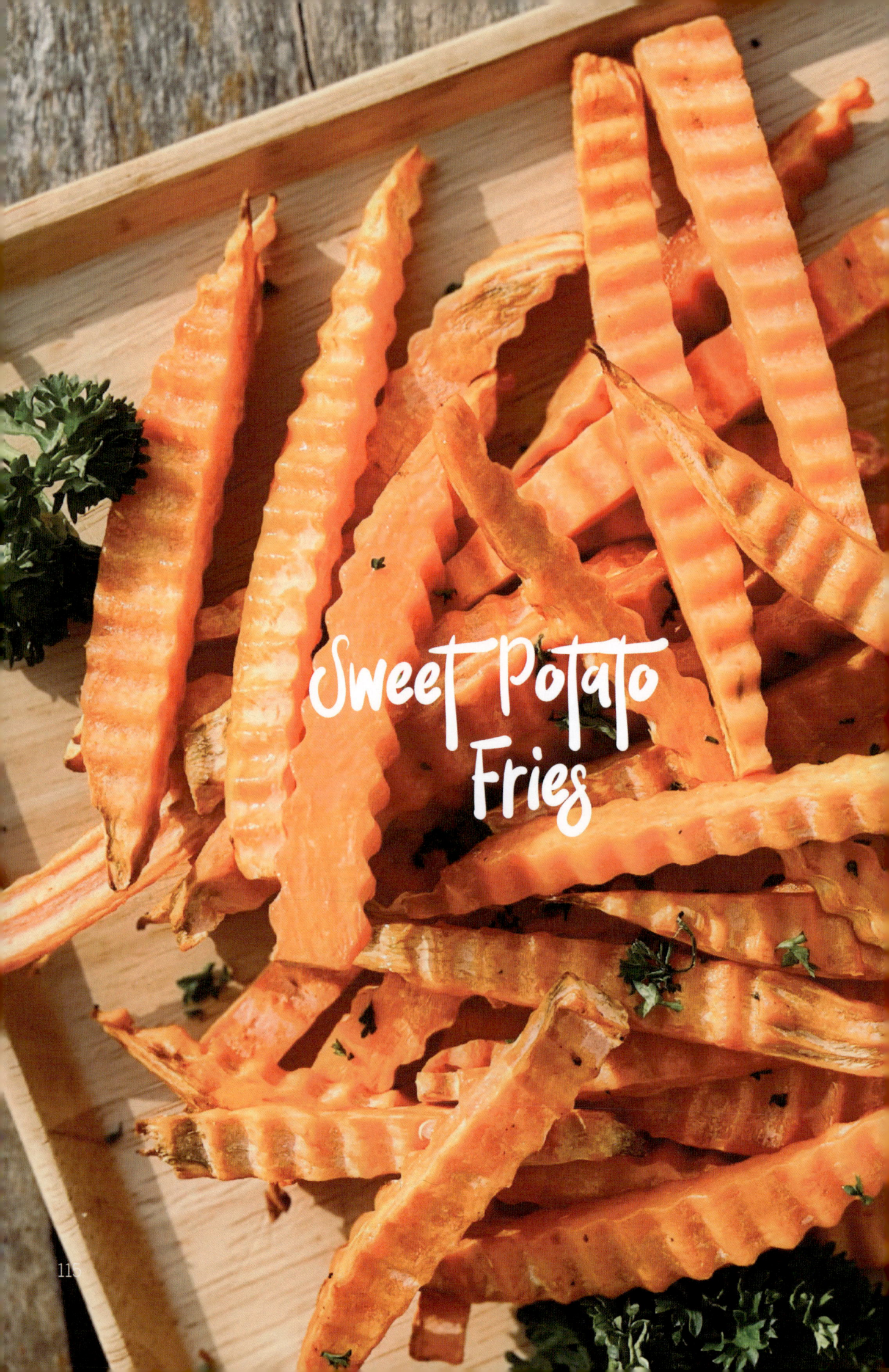

Sweet Potato Fries

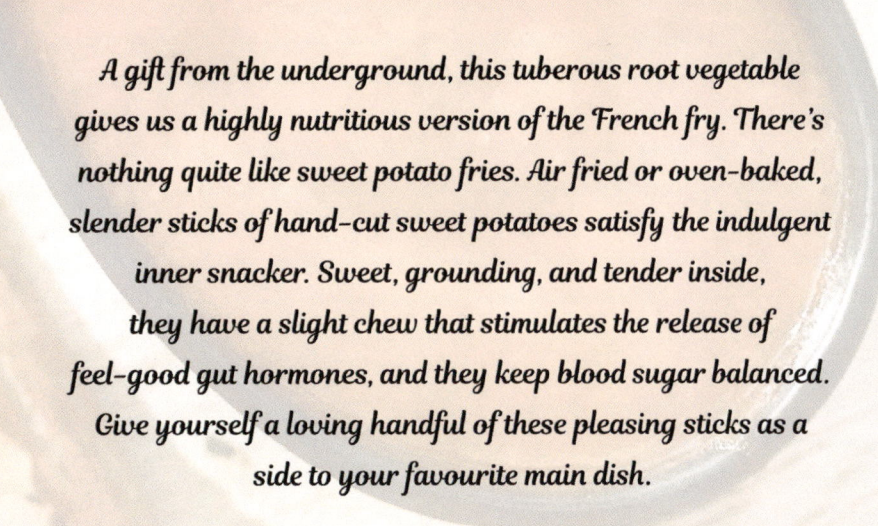

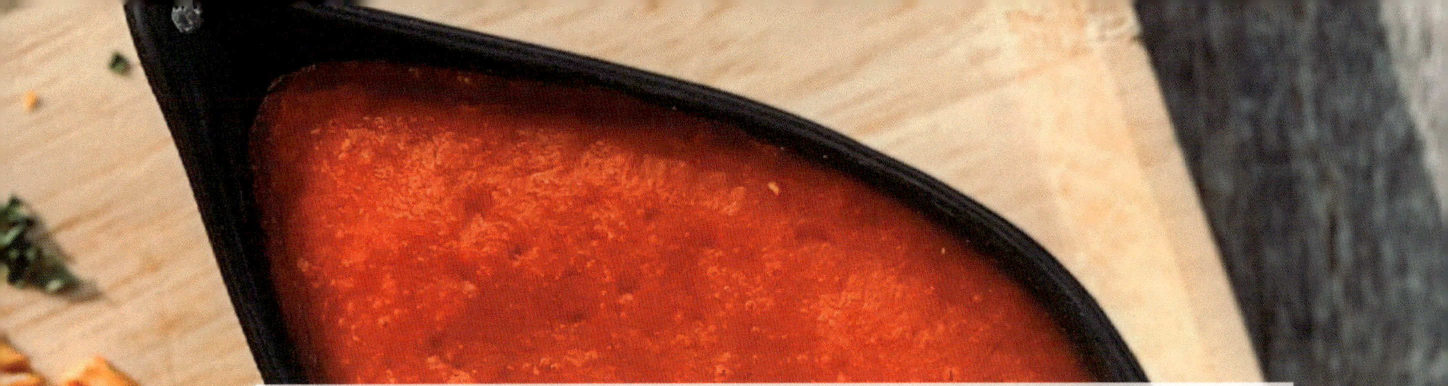

A gift from the underground, this tuberous root vegetable gives us a highly nutritious version of the French fry. There's nothing quite like sweet potato fries. Air fried or oven-baked, slender sticks of hand-cut sweet potatoes satisfy the indulgent inner snacker. Sweet, grounding, and tender inside, they have a slight chew that stimulates the release of feel-good gut hormones, and they keep blood sugar balanced. Give yourself a loving handful of these pleasing sticks as a side to your favourite main dish.

INGREDIENTS

1 Medium-sized sweet potato
1 tsp Olive oil
Pinch of Himalayan salt

INSTRUCTIONS

Cut the sweet potato lengthwise into fries. Cutting them into uniform sticks will ensure they cook evenly. In a large bowl, toss them lightly in the olive oil. Sprinkle with salt. Put the sweet potato sticks in an air fryer or oven. Bake at 200°C for 15 minutes, and toss them halfway through cooking.

Serving Size: 1 batch
Preparation Time: 20 minutes

Meaty and marvellous, roasted chickpeas contain a timeless essence of natural, nutritive power. Cumin and paprika pair to enhance a warming and grounding effect, and olive oil invites them all to dance.

INGREDIENTS

1 tbsp Olive oil

100 gr Pre-soaked and boiled (or canned) chickpeas

¼ tsp Cumin powder

¼ tsp Smoked paprika

Pinch of Himalayan salt

INSTRUCTIONS

Heat 1 tbsp of olive oil in a pan, add the chickpeas, spices, and salt. Roast in the pan evenly for about 2 minutes.

Serving Size: 1 batch
Preparation Time: 10 minutes

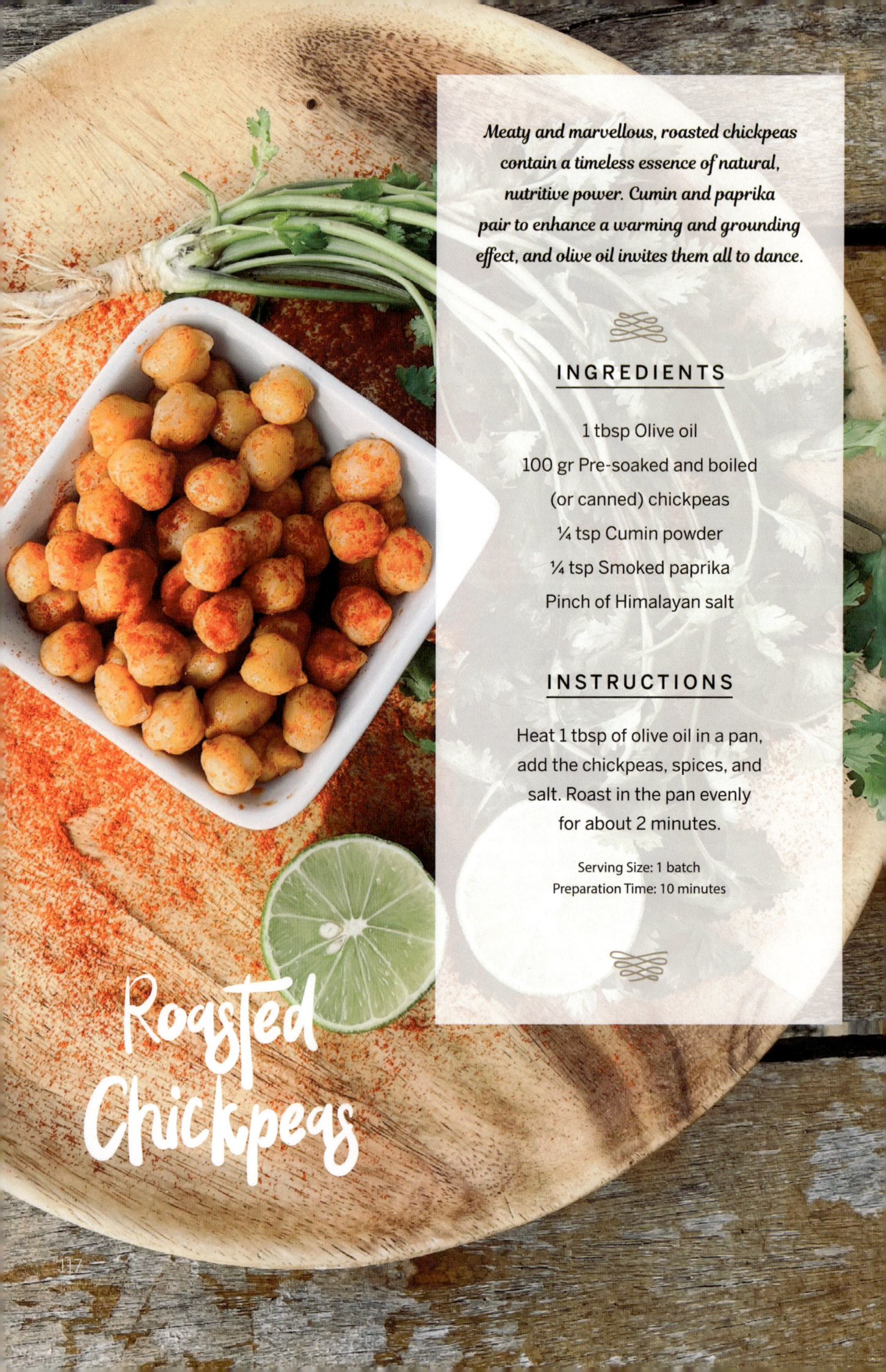

Roasted Chickpeas

A kiss of the Dark Goddess, the Earth Mother makes her appearance here in luxurious depths of rich and salty sweetness. Add the glistening power of inky magic to steamed veggies, exotic salads and used as a bewitching dipping sauce.

INGREDIENTS

½ cup Soy sauce

½ cup Water

30 gr Coconut sugar paste

1 tbsp Sesame oil

4 tbsp Apple cider vinegar

INSTRUCTIONS

Mix all ingredients in a big bowl and whisk until combined.

Serving Size: 1 batch
Preparation Time: 10 minutes

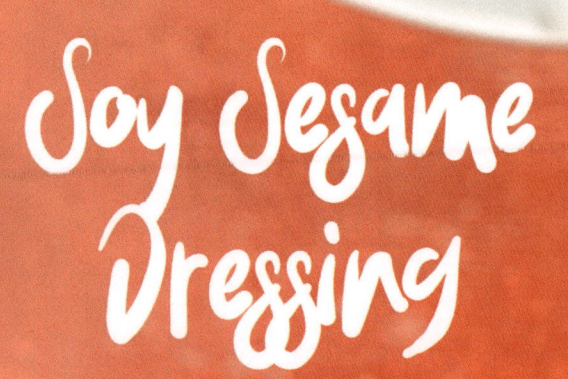

Soy Sesame Dressing

Ginger Lemon Tahini

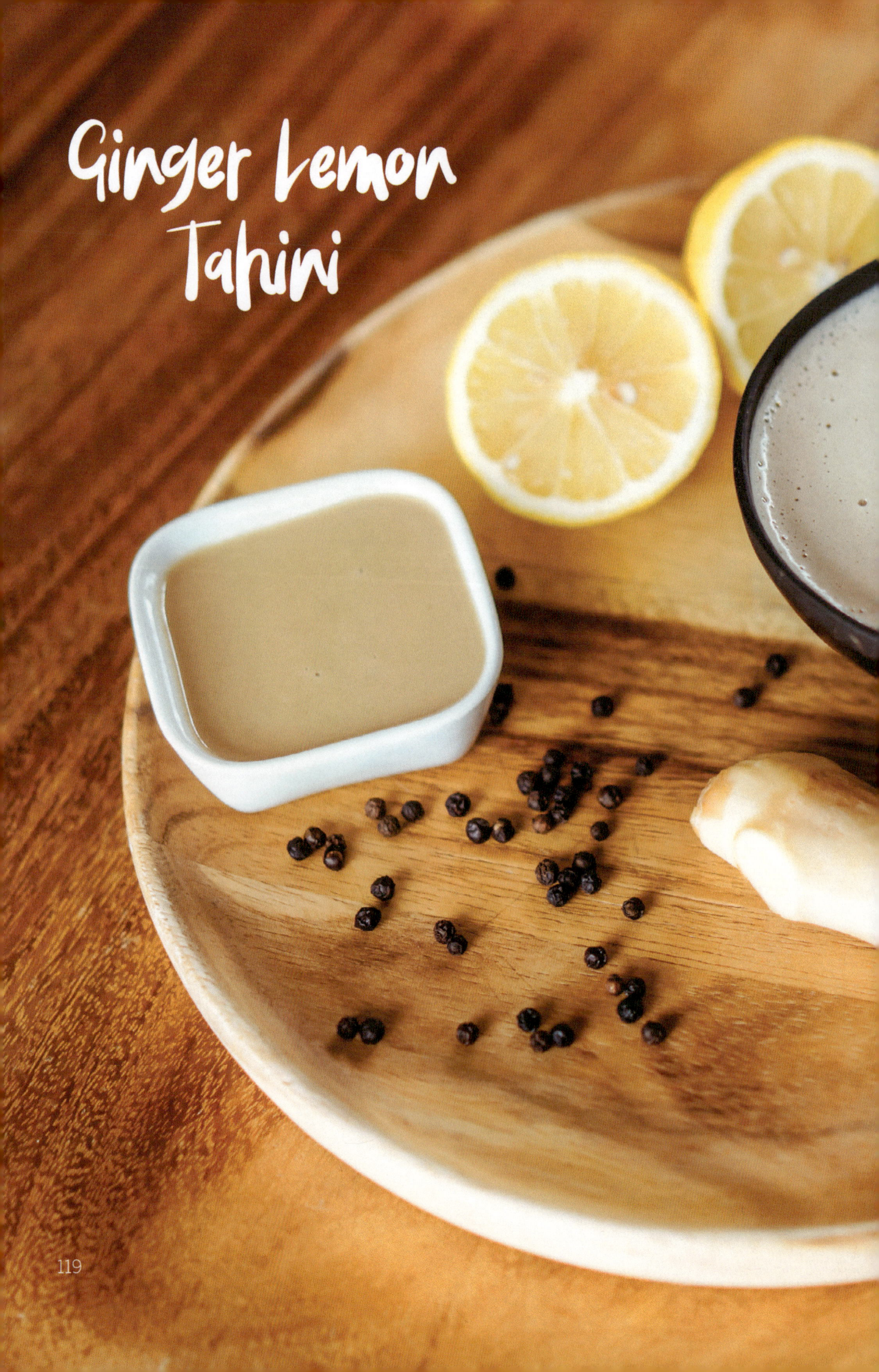

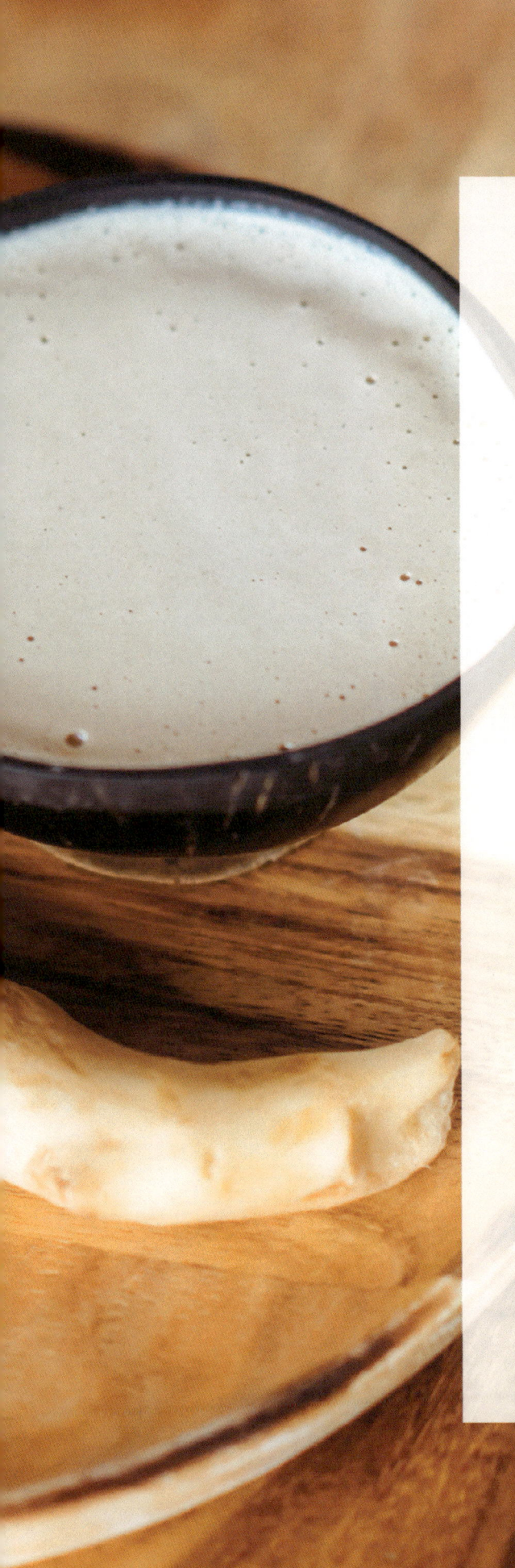

Only a trio made in the cosmos could be this good, but this one has a pure earth-made source. Rich, creamy tahini mellows out ginger's heat and lemon lends its citrusy kiss. Cast lashings of this dressing on a bed of fresh greens.

INGREDIENTS

2½ cups Tahini

2 tbsp Chopped ginger

⅔ cup Lemon juice

2 tsp Himalayan salt

1 tsp Black pepper

3½ cups Water

INSTRUCTIONS

Blend all ingredients in a high-speed blender until smooth. Store in an airtight container and refrigerate for up to 3 days.

Serving Size: 1 batch
Preparation Time: 10 minutes

A taste of sun-drunk mango with a hint of fragrant kaffir lime and tangy vinegar douse any salad or sandwich with sweet, drippy love. Smother this citrusy-sugar fusion recklessly, and discover how delicious abundance tastes.

INGREDIENTS

500 gr Mango

50 gr Coconut sugar paste

8 tbsp Apple cider vinegar

10 – 12 Kaffir lime leaves

½ tbsp Himalayan salt

INSTRUCTIONS

Put all ingredients in a high-speed blender and blend until smooth. Store in an airtight container and refrigerate for up to 3 days.

Serving Size: 1 batch
Preparation Time: 10 minutes

Mango & Kaffir Lime

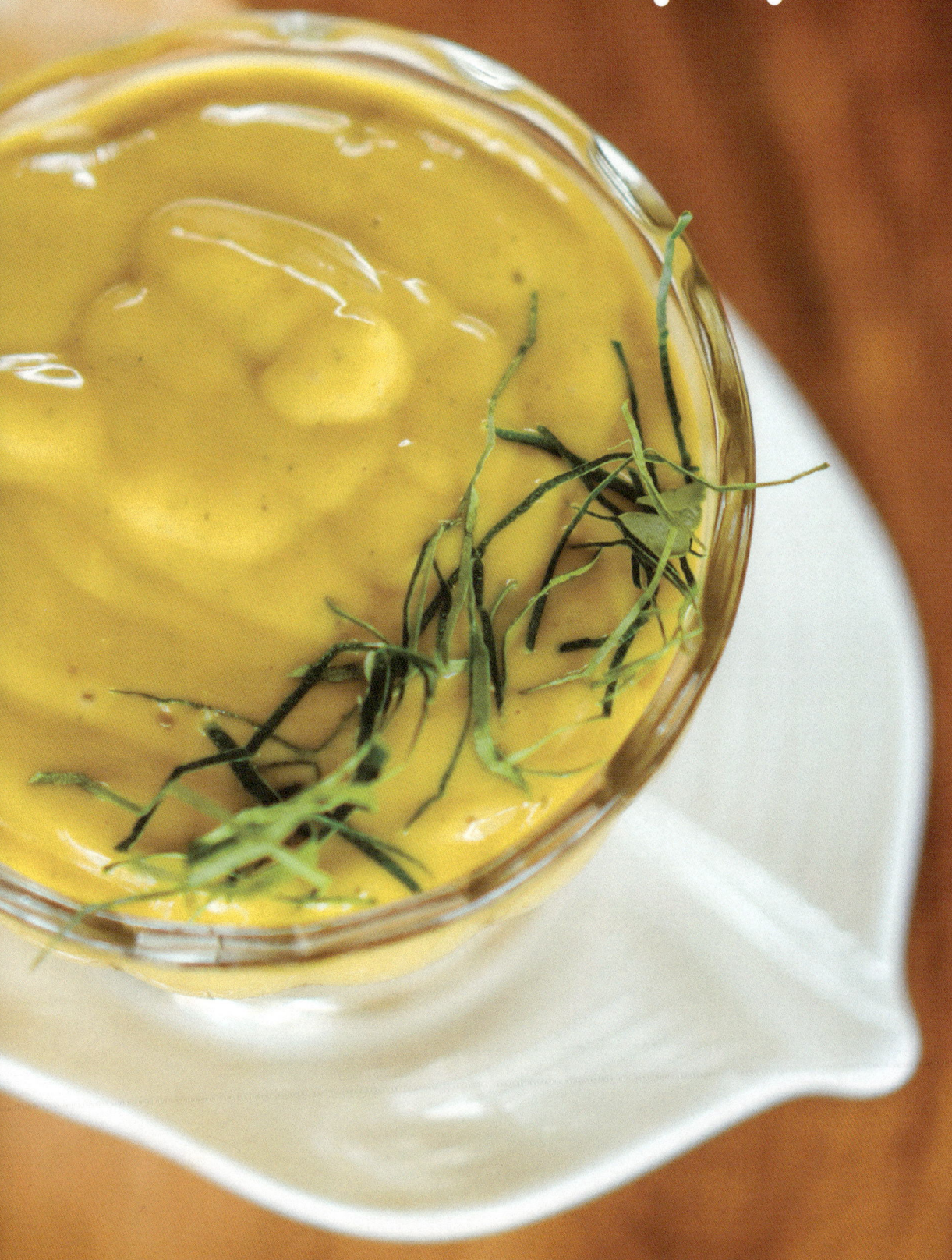

Light, tangy, and fragrant, this mélange of flavours extracts the best of kale and gives it new, lifted life. A salty, citrus kiss makes this pesto spread a delightful addition to raw cauliflower rice or other salad creation.

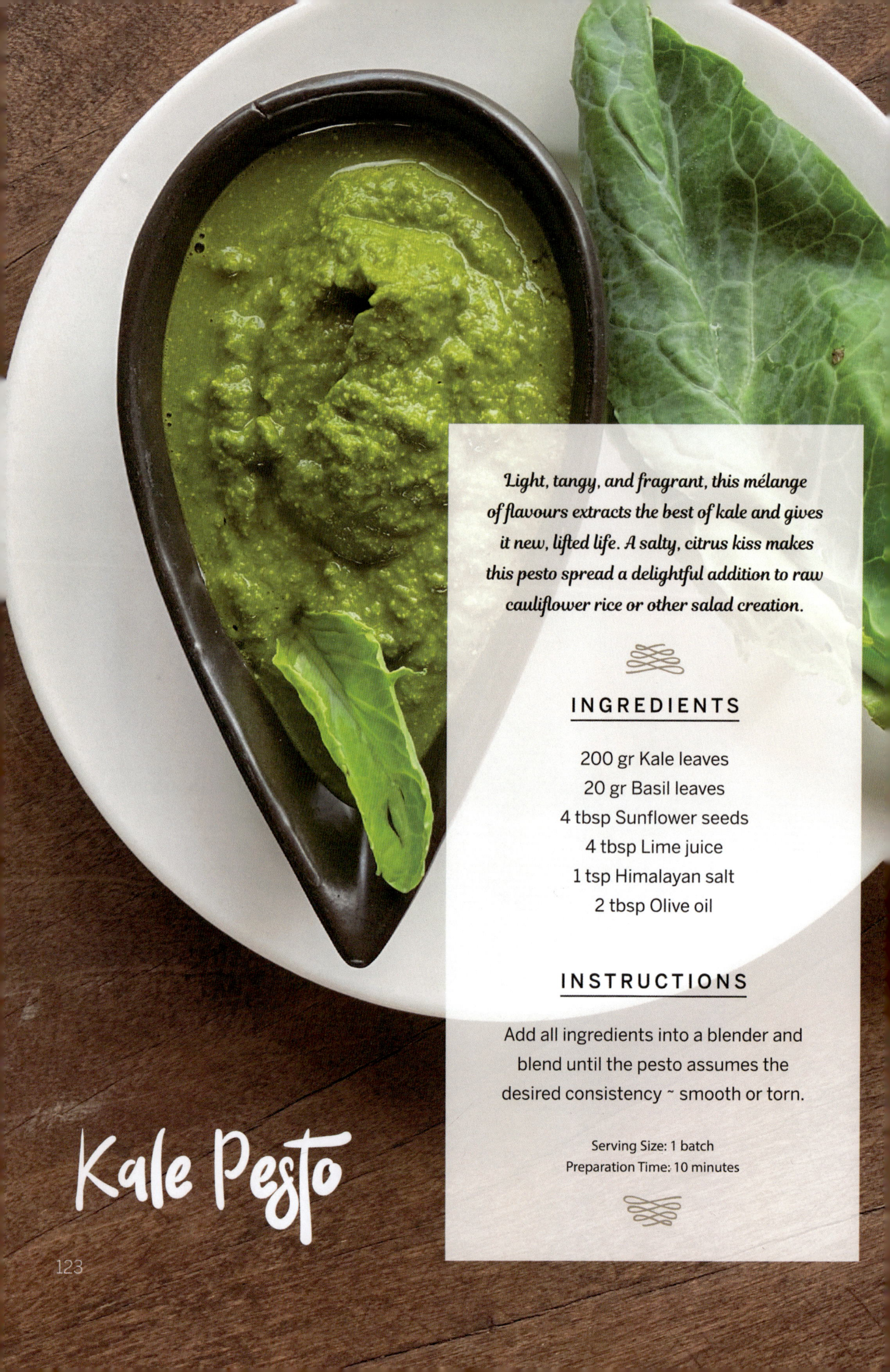

INGREDIENTS

200 gr Kale leaves
20 gr Basil leaves
4 tbsp Sunflower seeds
4 tbsp Lime juice
1 tsp Himalayan salt
2 tbsp Olive oil

INSTRUCTIONS

Add all ingredients into a blender and blend until the pesto assumes the desired consistency ~ smooth or torn.

Serving Size: 1 batch
Preparation Time: 10 minutes

Kale Pesto

Roasty Tomatoes

INGREDIENTS

200 gr Juicy cherry tomatoes
¼ cup Olive oil
5 bulbs Garlic, finely chopped
2 tsp Dried oregano
Sprinkle of Himalayan salt

INSTRUCTIONS

Halve and mix the tomatoes with the rest of the ingredients. Dehydrate using only the tray and not the sheet, at 40°C for 3 to 4 hours until dry and crispy. If oven baking, use extremely low heat to dehydrate for about half an hour, or until crispy. Add a chewy zest to your favourite dishes, store extras in an airtight container in the fridge for up to one week.

Serving Size: 1 batch
Preparation Time: 4 hours

Sweet, drippy tomato ketchup gets its pungent kick from apple cider vinegar, rich in beneficial bacteria. Coconut shows up again with a natural sweetness that gives ketchup its crave-worthy quality. Add a lashing or two of this lip-smacking sauce to your homemade burgers or for dunking Sweet Potato Fries.

INGREDIENTS

3 kg Large tomatoes

¾ cup Apple cider vinegar

300 gr Coconut sugar paste

5 tbsp Paprika powder

2 tbsp Himalayan salt

1 tbsp Guar gum

INSTRUCTIONS

Cut the tomatoes into big chunks and blend in a high-speed blender. Add the vinegar, coconut sugar paste, paprika powder, and salt, and blend until smooth. Transfer the mixture into a pot and cook on high heat, uncovered, until the mixture reduces by half and thickens. Add the guar gum and blend the mixture again for about 20 seconds. Transfer the ketchup into a jar and allow it to cool completely before serving.

Serving Size: 1 batch
Preparation Time: 1 hour

Tomato Ketchup

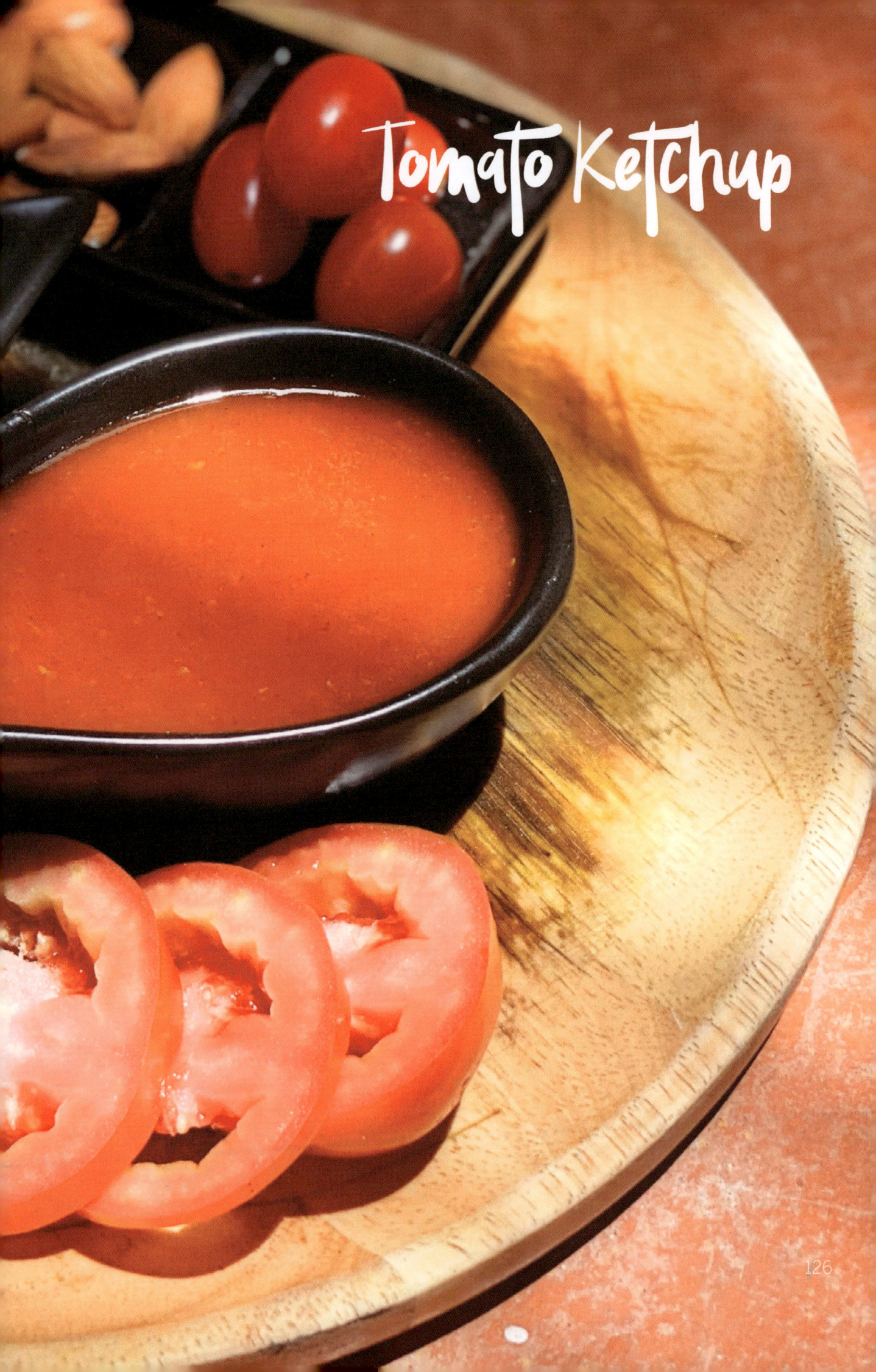

Cashew Cheese

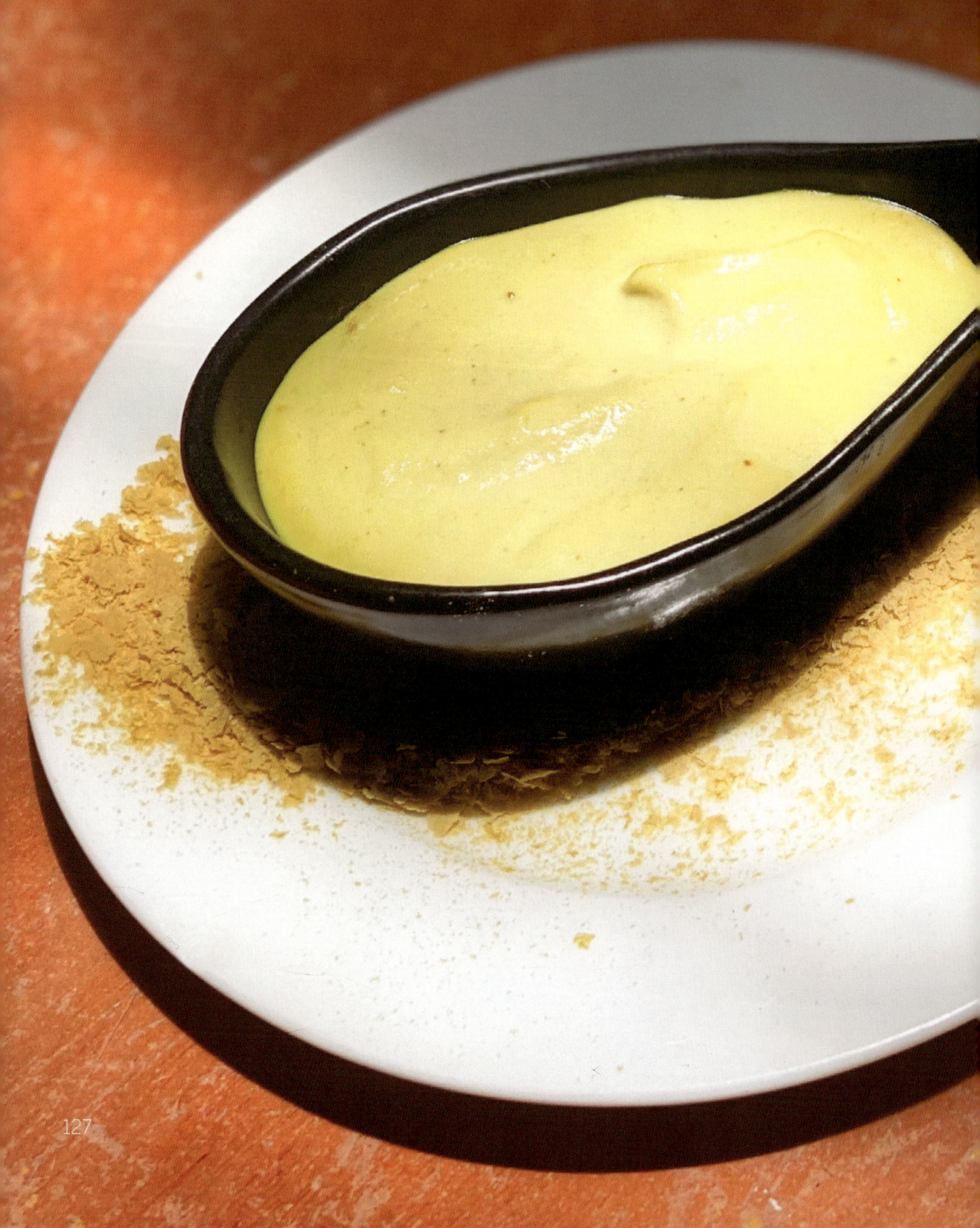

Drizzled or lazily smothered over Raw Trinity Tacos or other sensations, cashew cheese is redolent of wild, ancestral life. Turmeric and nutritional yeast mingle in perfect proportion to kick up the tangy pungent flavour and restore taste buds' intuitive intelligence. This isn't just a better cheese; it's the only cheese worthy of our tongues.

INGREDIENTS

500 gr Cashew nuts, soaked overnight

5 tbsp Nutritional yeast

1 tsp Turmeric powder

1 tsp Himalayan salt

1½ cups Water

INSTRUCTIONS

Soak the cashew nuts overnight or for at least four hours before proceeding. Drain and rinse the cashew nuts and transfer them to a high-speed blender with the remaining ingredients. Blend until completely smooth.

Serving Size: 1 batch
Preparation Time: 1 day

Crunchy, warming, and teeming with earthy essence. Sauerkraut is a gift for the belly because it's loaded with probiotics that help clean up and clear out. Finger-pick this slaw, add to a beetroot burger, or your favorite dish for extra sensation.

INGREDIENTS

1 large Purple cabbage

½ tbsp Himalayan salt

20 gr Ginger root

20 gr Coriander leaf

1½ cups Water

INSTRUCTIONS

Thinly slice the cabbage and put into a large bowl with the salt. Using your hands, massage the cabbage and the salt for about 10 to 15 minutes until it has a soft texture and has released a substantial amount of liquid. Chop the ginger root and coriander leaf and add to the cabbage. Transfer to a 1 litre glass jar, add water and close the lid tightly. Store at room temperature for three days to allow the fermentation process to occur.

Serving Size: 1 batch
Preparation Time: 3 days

Purple Sauerkraut

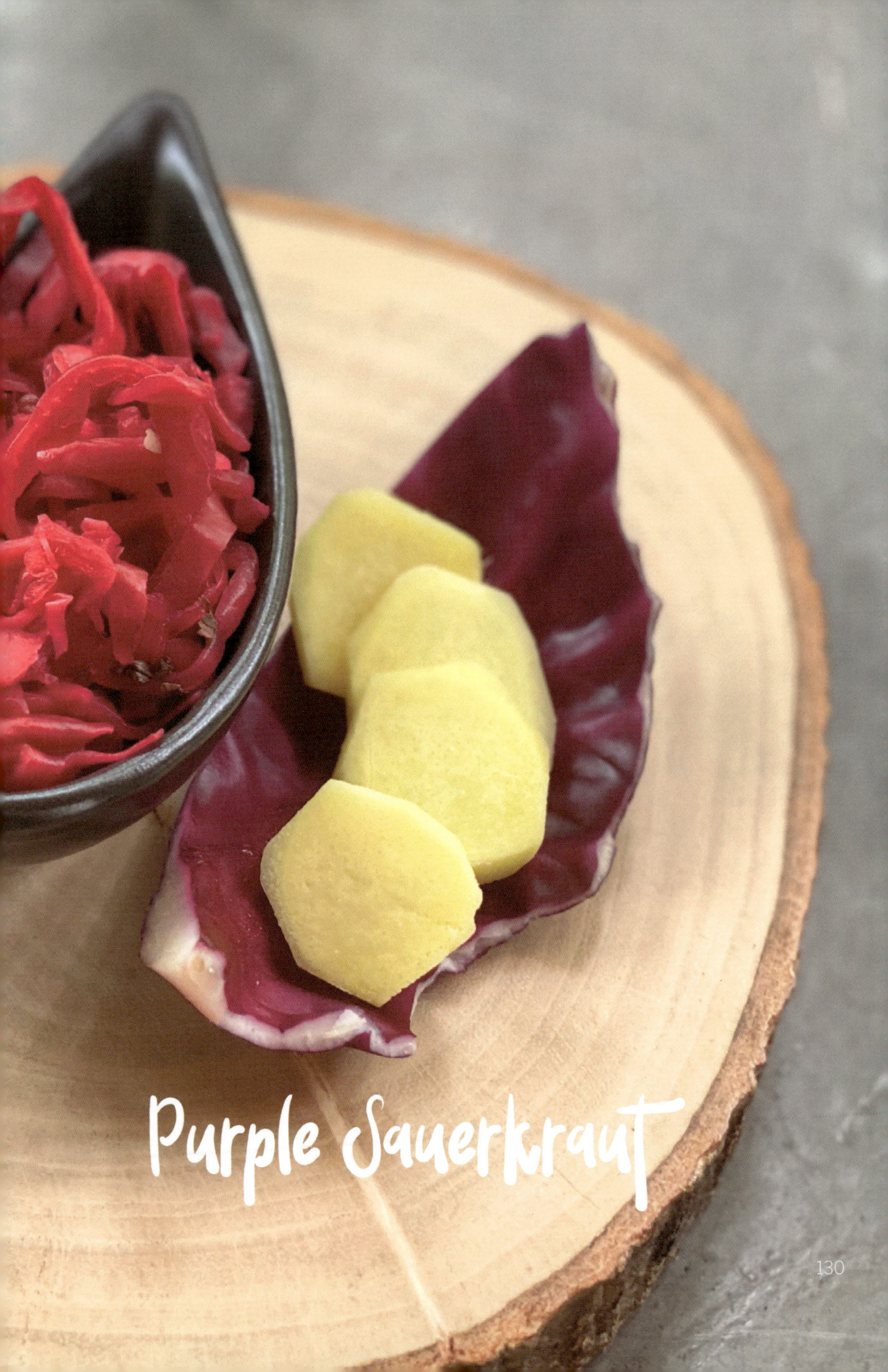

Vegan Parmesan

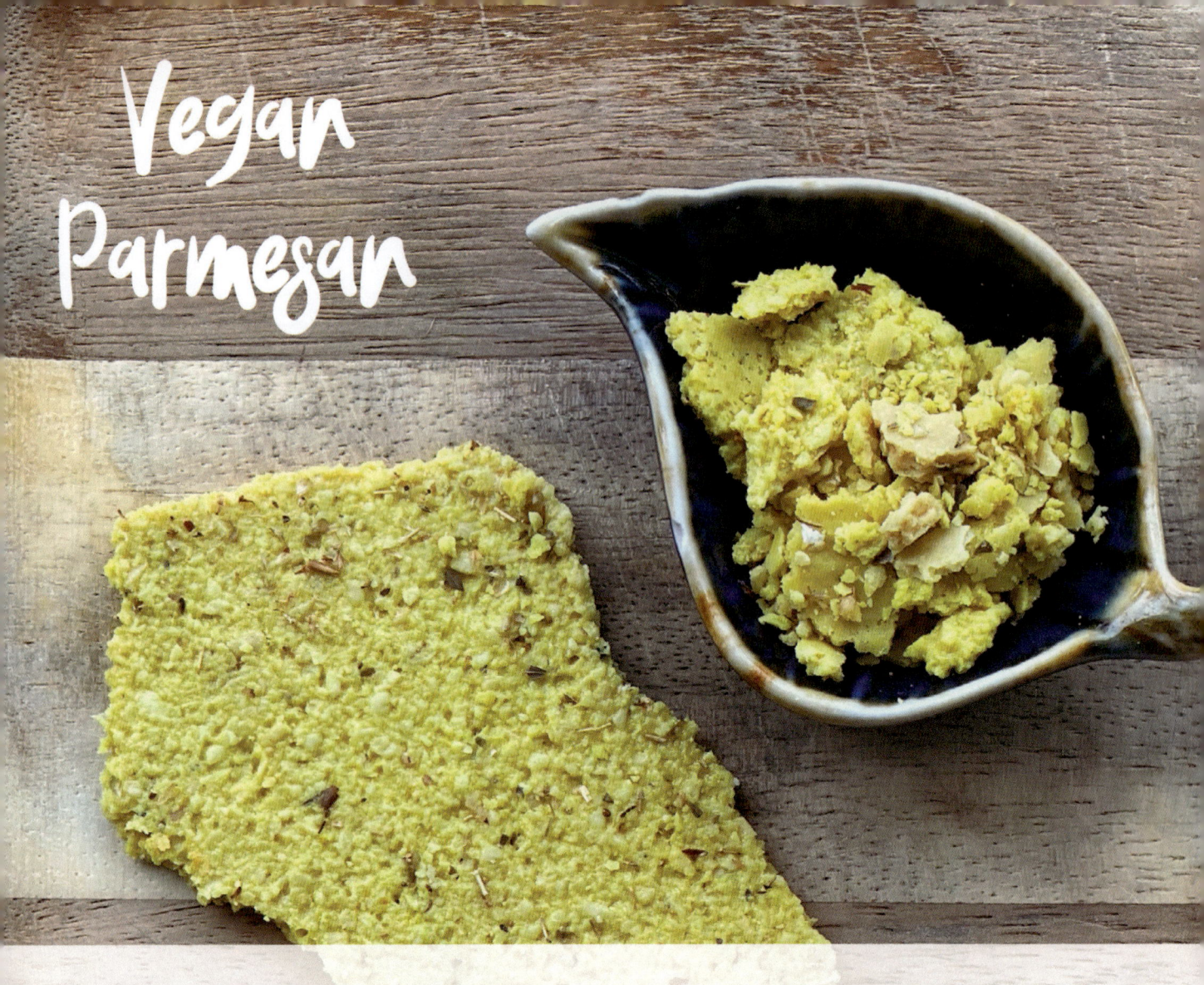

Tangy, mouthwatering, plant-based parmesan is a luscious topping for salads, pastas, steamed veggies, and more.

INGREDIENTS

300 gr Cashew nuts, soaked overnight

5 tbsp Nutritional yeast

2 tsp Dried oregano

2 tsp Himalayan salt

⅔ cup Fresh water

Juice of 2 Limes

Pinch of Turmeric powder

INSTRUCTIONS

Rinse the cashews well, soak overnight, wash thoroughly and mix with the rest of the ingredients in a high-speed blender. Transfer the mixture onto dehydrator trays fitted with parchment paper, and spread thin into ¼ inch layers. Score into the preferred shape and size using a cutter or knife. Then, set the dehydrator at 45°C and dehydrate for about 4 hours. Remove the cheese from the parchment paper and turn it over directly onto the tray to dehydrate for an additional 4 hours, or until the parmesan is completely dry and crispy.

Serving Size: 1 batch
Preparation Time: 1½ day

Cashew Basil Pesto

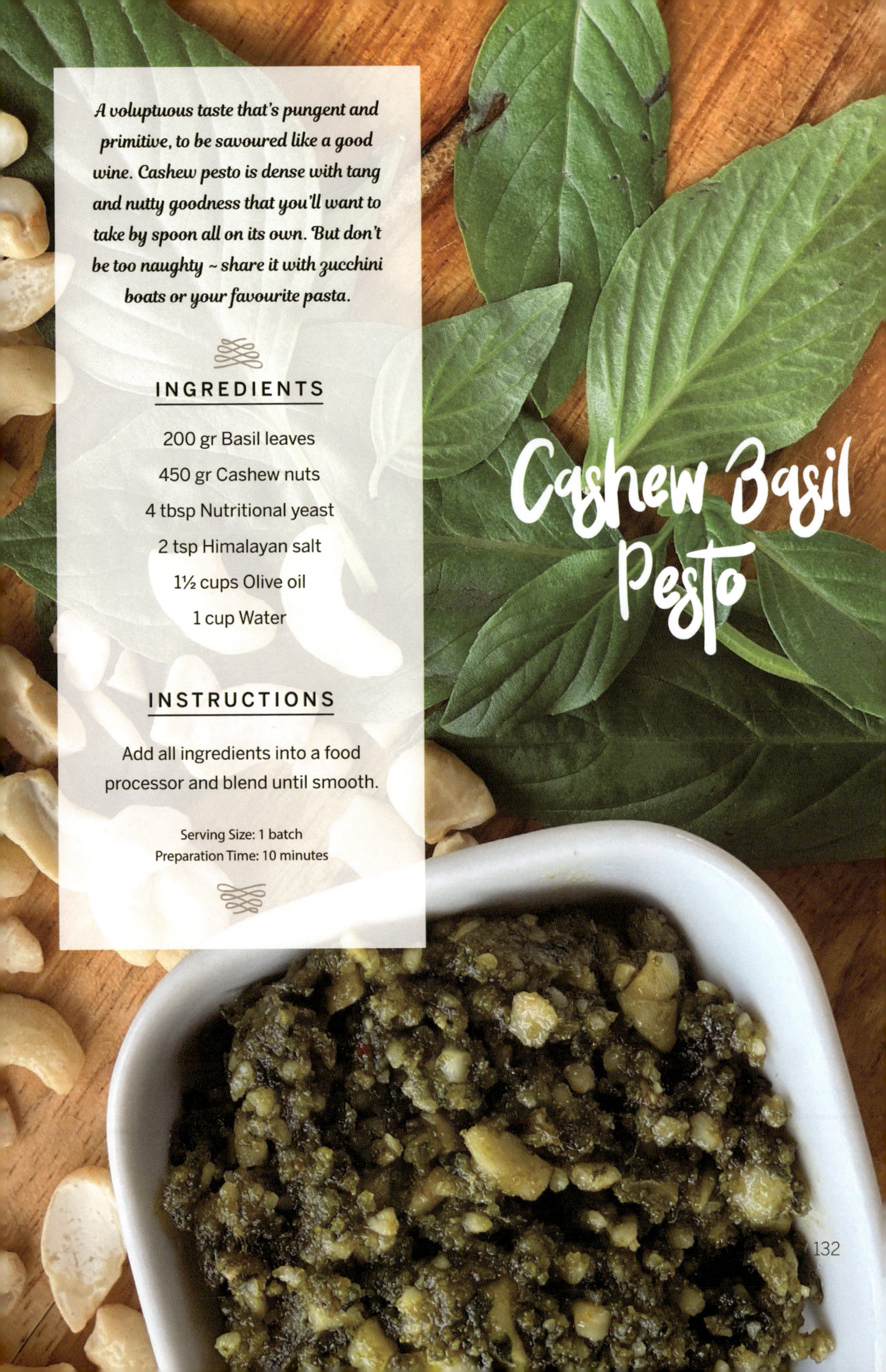

A voluptuous taste that's pungent and primitive, to be savoured like a good wine. Cashew pesto is dense with tang and nutty goodness that you'll want to take by spoon all on its own. But don't be too naughty ~ share it with zucchini boats or your favourite pasta.

INGREDIENTS

200 gr Basil leaves

450 gr Cashew nuts

4 tbsp Nutritional yeast

2 tsp Himalayan salt

1½ cups Olive oil

1 cup Water

INSTRUCTIONS

Add all ingredients into a food processor and blend until smooth.

Serving Size: 1 batch
Preparation Time: 10 minutes

Caesar Dressing

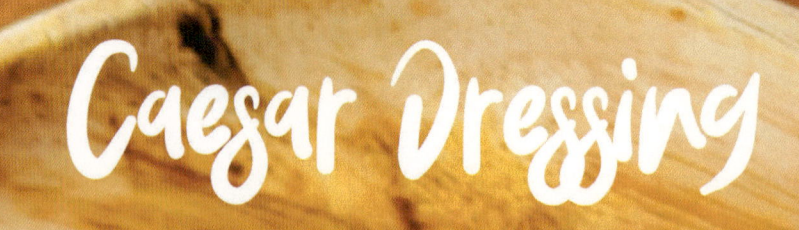

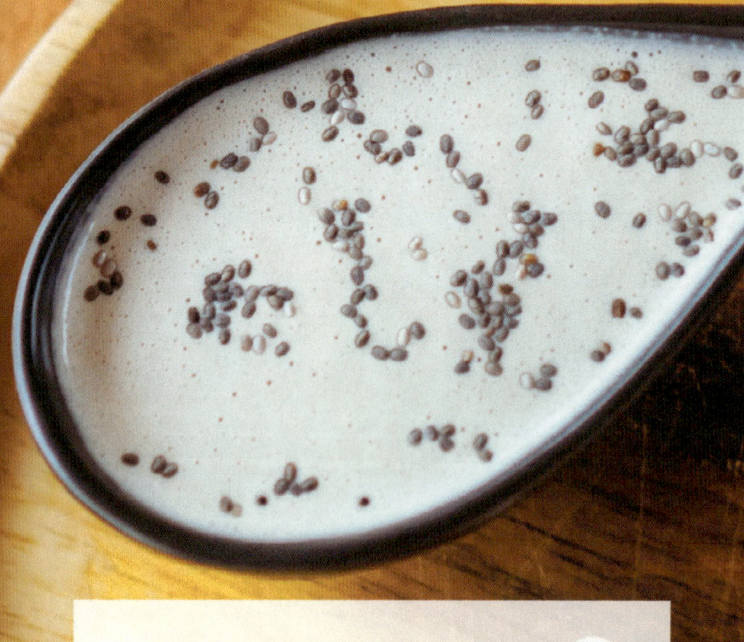

INGREDIENTS

100 gr Cashew nuts, soaked overnight

1 tsp Himalayan salt

¼ tsp Black pepper

1 tbsp Chia seeds (not soaked)

1⅓ cup Water or coconut water

½ Clove of garlic

INSTRUCTIONS

Rinse the cashews well and soak overnight. Wash thoroughly and mix with the rest of the ingredients in a high-speed blender until smooth and creamy.

Serving Size: 1 batch
Preparation Time: 1 day

Coconut Bacon

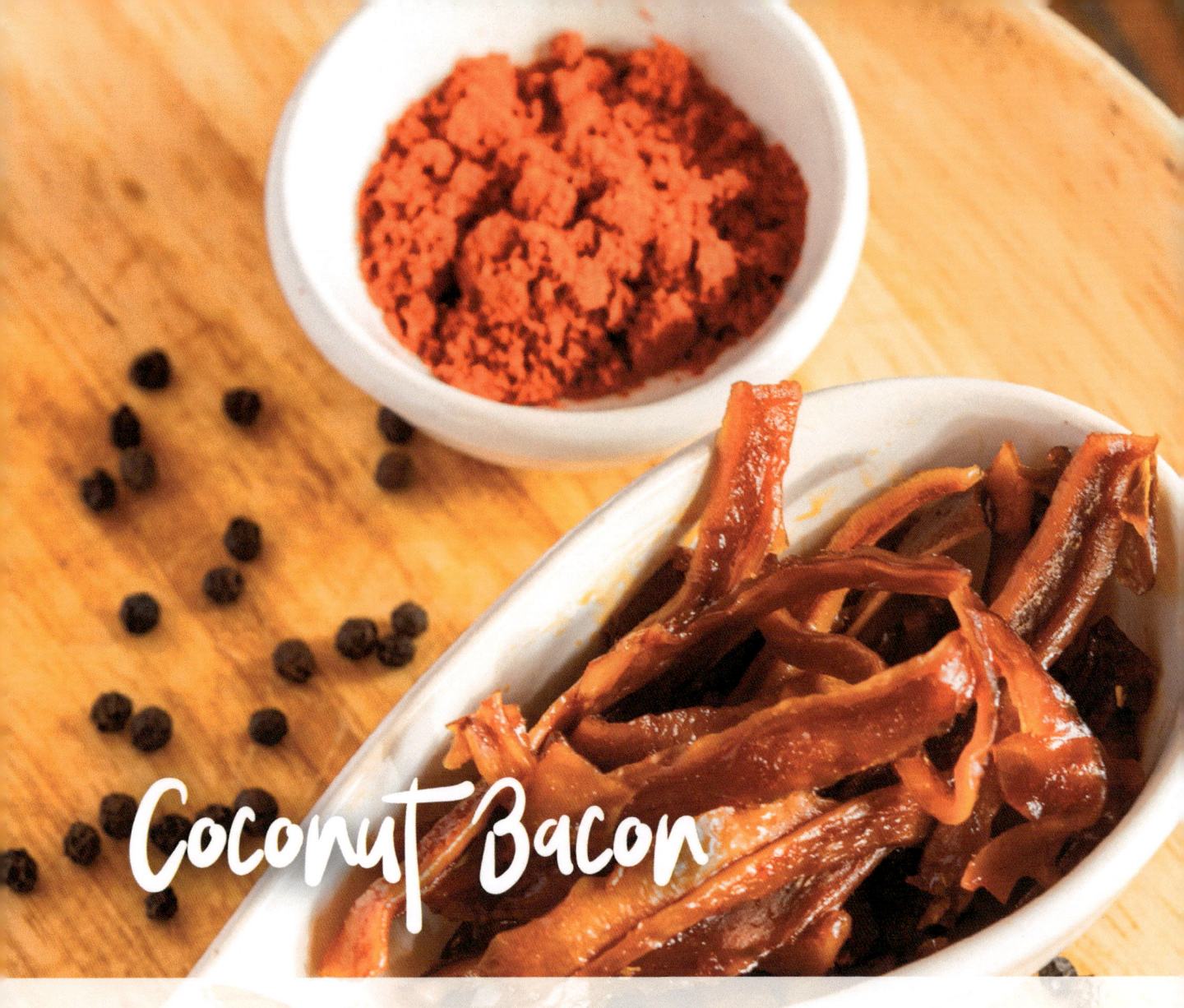

INGREDIENTS

20 gr Fresh or frozen coconut meat

15 ml Sesame oil

30 ml Soy sauce (or gluten-free soy)

1 tsp Paprika

15 ml Coconut syrup

½ tsp Liquid smoke - optional

1 pinch Himalayan salt

½ tsp Black pepper

INSTRUCTIONS

Cut the coconut meat into finger-sized strips and set aside while mixing all the other ingredients. When your mixture is completely dissolved, add the coconut and rest to marinate. Spread the strips and paste onto a dehydrator tray and dehydrate at 40°C for 2 hours or until completely dry. To oven-dry, use lowest heat (you can use a wooden spoon to keep the door ajar) and slow bake about half an hour, until crispy. If you can't access coconut, you can switch out with the smokey goodness of roasted eggplant.

Serving Size: 1 batch
Preparation Time: 2½ hours

ACKNOWLEDGMENTS

Project Manager
Daliah Barkan

Project Assistant
Rebecca Haas

Editor
Jade Richardson

Creative Writer
Colleen Thornton

Graphic Designer
Hila Gersztenkorn
Vincenzo Vigliarolo

Recipe Supervision & Food Presentation
Chef Sandeep Painuli

Cover Design
Vincenzo Vigliarolo

Photography
Marco Reez
Ben Minot
Elsa Pehe
Ali Iua
Alice Sudos
Oom Chaowanapreecha

Models
Nabi Tang
Doris Kemptner
Passalak Supasiripisarn 'Dream'
Mari Heart
Joanna Cambrand
Vanessa Jose
Deborah Vilardi
Bryce Draper

**Thank you to all additional members of
our island community featured in the book.**

Thank you all for making this happen!

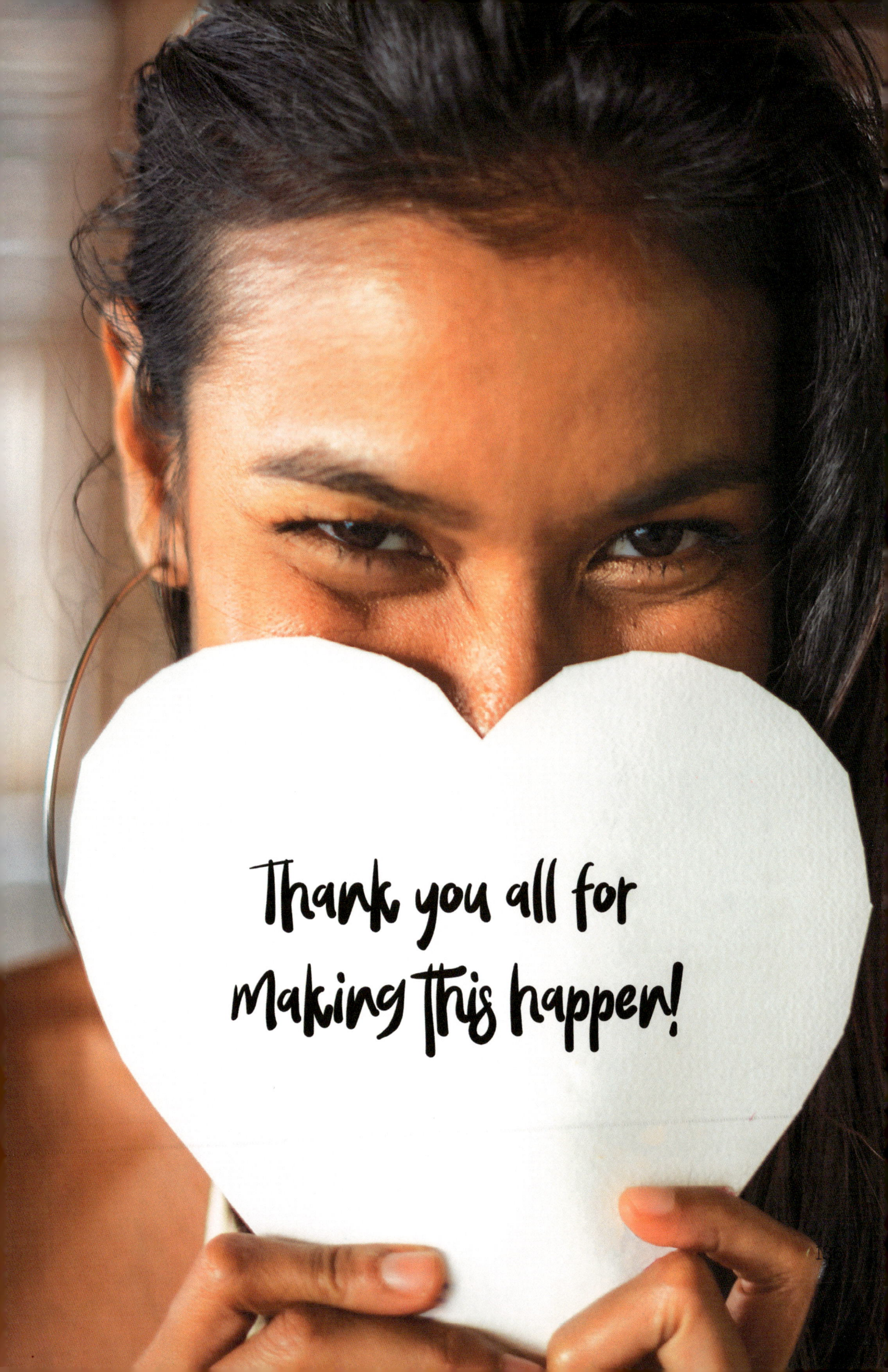

NOTES

NOTES

NOTES

NOTES

Printed in Great Britain
by Amazon